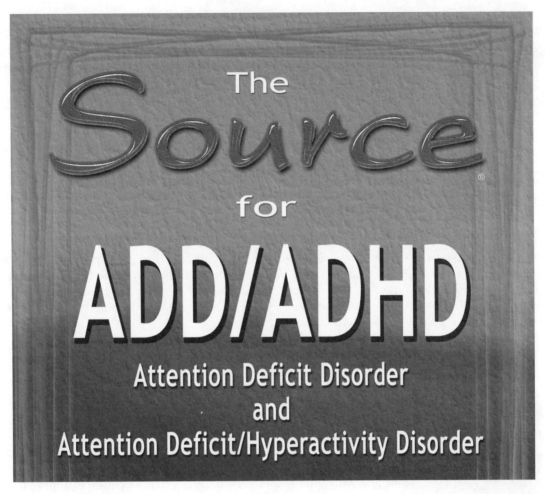

The *Source* for
ADD/ADHD

Attention Deficit Disorder
and
Attention Deficit/Hyperactivity Disorder

Gail J. Richard
Joy L. Russell

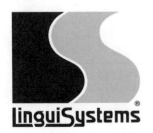

LinguiSystems®

| Skill Area: | ADD/ADHD |
| Ages: | All Ages |

LinguiSystems, Inc.
3100 4th Avenue
East Moline, IL 61244-9700

800-776-4332

FAX: 800-577-4555
E-mail: service@linguisystems.com
Web: linguisystems.com

Printed in the U.S.A.

ISBN 0-7606-0380-4

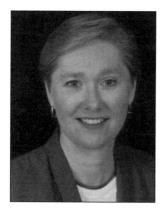

Gail J. Richard, Ph.D., CCC-SLP, is a professor and Acting Chair in the Department of Communication Disorders & Sciences at Eastern Illinois University in Charleston, Illinois. She teaches undergraduate and graduate courses and serves as a clinical supervisor for diagnostic and clinical practicum experiences. Gail enjoys the challenges presented in childhood developmental language disorders, such as autistic spectrum disorders, language processing, language-learning disabilities, and selective mutism. Prior to her 20 years at Eastern, Gail's professional experience included working as a public school speech clinician and in a diagnostic/therapeutic preschool setting. She consults extensively with other professionals, teachers, parents, and school districts to assist in providing educational programming suggestions for children with special needs. Gail also presents numerous workshops around the country, sharing her practical clinical knowledge with audiences.

This is Gail's sixth book in LinguiSystems' *Source®* Series. Previous publications with LinguiSystems include *The Source for Autism*, *The Source for Treatment Methodologies in Autism*, and *The Source for Processing Disorders*. She is also the co-author of *The Source for Syndromes* and *The Source for Syndromes 2* with Debra Reichert Hoge, and *Language Processing Test-Revised* and *Language Processing Kit* with Mary Anne Hanner.

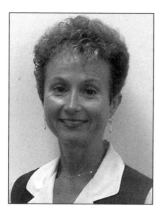

Joy L. Russell, M.S. in Education, is the Executive Administrator for the Regional Office of Education in Charleston, Illinois, where she is in charge of professional development for educators and administrations in a seven county area. Joy also works part-time at Eastern Illinois University in the Department of Special Education as an instructor for both graduate and undergraduate courses. Her experience includes 11 years as a special education teacher in K-12, working with children who had a variety of disabilities, including learning disorders, social-emotional disorders, autism, traumatic brain injury, and various degrees of mental impairment. Joy moved from the classroom to an administrative position with the Eastern Illinois Area of Special Education as Technical Assistants Coordinator. In that capacity she organized staffings; team meetings; and child, parent, and professional consultations. Joy also served as a resource in the provision of appropriate educational programs for students with special needs. This is Joy's first publication with LinguiSystems.

Dedication

To Alex Russell, with deepest love and respect; In life you served as Joy's constant support, objective critic, and exemplified a true "joie de vivre"! You are missed greatly by all the individuals whose lives you touched in your too-short time with us on Earth.

Table of Contents

Chapter 1

Introduction

Professionals working with children are increasingly faced with a diagnosis of Attention Deficit Disorder (ADD) and Attention Deficit/Hyperactivity Disorder (ADD/ADHD). The questions start, and the frustration builds.

- What is the disorder?
- What do I do to help children who have it?
- What am I going to do to help other professionals and parents understand the disorder?
- How can I help this child function productively in other environments?
- Is there a clear resource to guide my efforts?

There is a great deal of information available to parents and professionals in regard to ADD/ADHD. The challenge becomes how to pull it all together in a succinct, coherent way that clears up foggy concepts. Many times impressions are based on stories or personal experiences, which might present a one-sided perspective of ADD/ADHD. Let's work through a few of the common false impressions regarding the disorder.

Myths and Realities

There are many myths that swirl around the professional arena when discussing ADD/ADHD. This section will present some of the major myths, followed by the reality as it exists presently. The myths that are addressed include the following:

1. Children will outgrow ADD/ADHD.
2. Hyperactivity is a component of all children with attention deficit disorders.
3. Diagnosis is made by a physician.
4. ADD/ADHD occurs in males.
5. Diagnosis for ADD/ADHD occurs before second grade or in primary elementary school.
6. It's not ADD/ADHD; it's poor effort and work habits.

7. ADD/ADHD is over diagnosed; teachers don't want active learners.

8. ADD/ADHD is caused by poor diet, discipline, etc.

9. Allergies cause ADD/ADHD.

10. Medication is not necessary in ADD/ADHD.

11. Medication causes more problems than it helps in ADD/ADHD.

12. Medication will take care of ADD/ADHD.

13. The disability of ADD/ADHD accounts for all the problems in these children.

14. If ADD/ADHD is diagnosed, the child must be classified under "Special Education" in the school system.

15. There is a set intervention that works for children with ADD/ADHD.

Myth:

Children will outgrow ADD/ADHD.

"My physician said not to worry. If we can survive until Leon reaches age 12, he should have outgrown the worst of it by then."

Reality:

80% of the children with ADD/ADHD will NOT grow out of the disorder. What can happen is that with time and maturity, many of these children learn to channel their excessive energy in a constructive way. They might appear to be "Type A" personalities or someone who is always on the go. The ADD/ADHD is still present; it is simply managed better. While many children's hyperactivity seems to abate, the inattentiveness and academic difficulties may continue. Teachers and parents might report that the problem is "going away," but the problems associated with ADD/ADHD could become more subtle. The child with ADD/ADHD might find ways to vent and control the hyperactivity component better, but other characteristics that negatively impact the ability to function effectively in the world are still present. The myth will be more fully addressed in Chapter 3, explaining the evolution of the disorder over the life span.

Myth:

Hyperactivity is a component of all children with attention deficit disorders.

"I can't believe Will was diagnosed with ADD/ADHD. He's never out of his desk or bouncing off the walls of my classroom."

Reality:

Not all children with ADD/ADHD present with extreme over-activity in their behavioral characteristics. The inability to pay attention isn't always physically obvious. A body doesn't have to be constantly moving around to indicate problems maintaining focus. The deficit in attention can appear to be a child who has his head down on the desk and is interpreted as sleepy or lazy. It could be the class clown who acts up to cover the embarrassment of not knowing what the teacher is talking about. It could also be the child who talks a mile a minute but never seems to say anything. Chapter 3 will discuss the characteristics of ADD/ADHD.

Myth:

Diagnosis is made by a physician.

"The doctor said not to worry about her. She's just active."

Reality:

Although ADD/ADHD is a disorder defined medically in *The Diagnostic and Statistical Manual of Mental Disorders, Fourth Edition* (2000), the best approach for diagnosis involves input from a team of individuals working with a child. Professionals in an education setting are more likely to observe the characteristics associated with ADD/ADHD. When multiple professionals are involved in delineating the characteristic profile which results in a diagnosis of ADD/ADHD, the greater the confidence in the accuracy of the label. The professional roles and responsibilities in diagnosis are discussed in Chapters 4 and 10.

Myth:

ADD/ADHD occurs in males.
"Teachers just aren't used to such an active girl who doesn't sit still."

Reality:

ADD/ADHD does occur with higher frequency in males than in females, but that doesn't mean that it doesn't occur in girls. The reality is that it isn't diagnosed as often in females because they might not exhibit the major behavioral issues that boys do. The female students are sometimes more astute in socially covering the characteristics so that the disability doesn't immediately come to the attention of teachers, parents, and other professionals. Chapter 5 addresses some of the research on gender differences with ADD/ADHD.

Myth:

Diagnosis for ADD/ADHD occurs before second grade or in primary elementary school.
"My son is in junior high. It's part of puberty, not ADD/ADHD."

Reality:

The age of the child at diagnosis tends to be a function of the severity of the disorder, rather than onset age. It is not unusual to diagnose ADD/ADHD during junior high, high school, and even adult years. There are many adults who fit the diagnostic criteria for ADD/ADHD but were never diagnosed. Children who are more intelligent can often compensate for problems associated with the disorder until things begin to snowball in higher academic grades. Suddenly they have multiple teachers and schedules to adjust to, and their difficulties blow up into overt, external problems that they can't control on their own. Information in Chapters 2, 3, and 4 addresses aspects of this myth.

Myth:

It's not ADD/ADHD; it's poor effort and work habits.
"There's nothing wrong with my kid. He just doesn't apply himself. He needs to work harder."

Reality:

Children are often blamed for legitimate disabilities. One of the characteristics of ADD/ADHD is an uneven achievement pattern across academic subjects and from day to day. Children with ADD/ADHD are often unable to sustain steady, consistent work. When a teacher or parent sees good work some of the time, she presumes a student is capable of performing at that level all the time. It's not fair to the child when professionals don't understand that one of the problems in ADD/ADHD is difficulty sustaining a level of work performance over a concentrated period of time. One of the main features of ADD/ADHD is trouble executing skills. Chapters 5 and 8 address this in more detail.

Myth:

ADD/ADHD is over diagnosed; teachers don't want active learners.
"That teacher refers everyone in her class for ADD/ADHD testing. She just can't cope with kids."

Reality:

The actual prevalence of ADD/ADHD varies widely based on assessment tools and procedures used to diagnose. Incidence figures estimate that between 3-10% of school age children are affected by ADD/ADHD. Most studies substantiate a 5% level of incidence, but many females are not diagnosed because the symptoms are evidenced in a more subtle way. It's also important to understand that a lone teacher cannot diagnose ADD/ADHD. The label requires a group process where the majority of team members are in agreement with the characteristic profile. Chapters 4 and 6 expand on aspects that deal with diagnostic issues of ADD/ADHD.

Myth:

ADD/ADHD is caused by poor diet, discipline, etc.
"Kenisha isn't hyperactive. She just drinks too much soda, eats the wrong stuff, and doesn't pay attention."

Reality:

While nutrition and diet can contribute to magnifying certain symptoms of ADD/ADHD, factors like too much sugar or poor discipline do not account for this disorder by themselves. Over 50% of children diagnosed with ADD/ADHD have a parent who also has the disability, diagnosed or not. Research is suggesting a genetic link in many cases, and neurological causes encoded in DNA that result in the observed deficits. Chapters 3 and 4 further address causes of ADD/ADHD, and Chapter 6 discusses dietary treatments.

Myth:

Allergies cause ADD/ADHD.
"The research says kids with ADD/ADHD have allergy problems. That's the cause of the ADD/ADHD."

Reality:

Children with ADD/ADHD are more prone to allergies, ear infections, and other mild medical problems. The coexistence of other disorders signals a pattern of subtle neurological differences that are part of the ADD/ADHD profile; however, the existence of other ailments does not mean they are the cause of ADD/ADHD. Correlation of other problems does not imply cause. Other possible ailments that co-occur with ADD/ADHD are discussed in Chapter 2.

Myth:

Medication is not necessary in ADD/ADHD.
"Allie might have ADD/ADHD, but she doesn't need medication.
She can learn to pay attention."

Reality:

ADD/ADHD is documented as a neurological difference within
the central nervous system, specifically the brainstem and cortex.
It is not a behavior problem that should be blamed on a child.
When a child has a neurological disorder, it is logical to explore
neurological treatment. Stimulant medication has been shown to
be effective in children, adolescents, and adults. It decreases
hyperactivity and impulsivity, while improving attention and concentration. Options in medical treatment are addressed more
fully in Chapter 6.

Myth:

Medication causes more problems than it helps in ADD/ADHD.
"Ritalin does bad things. I'll take my chances with the
ADD/ADHD by itself."

Reality:

Research has shown that adjustment problems to medication,
such as poor appetite, are generally short-term and re-adjust back
to normal levels within six months. Ritalin is a relatively safe
medication with minimal side effects when compared to the positive effects on attention and learning for many children. Any
medication can have side effects, and in some cases, long-term
detrimental effects have been documented. That's why careful
monitoring and communication are critical in ADD/ADHD.
Chapter 6 presents information on the pharmacological
recommendations for the disorder.

Myth:

Medication will take care of ADD/ADHD.
"I agreed to medication, but it hasn't helped at all. My child isn't doing any better in school."

Reality:

Medication does not cure the disability of ADD/ADHD. The symptoms become less severe, but medication doesn't "fix" the problem. A child with a strong personality, discipline challenges, and aggressive tendencies is not going to become a perfect angel in response to medication. The pharmacological intervention must be in combination with strong structure and support in the home and academic environments. Chapter 6 discusses the role of medication in more detail.

Myth:

The disability of ADD/ADHD accounts for all the problems in these children.
"They can't suspend him from school because he has ADD/ADHD. That's the reason he's fighting all the time."

Reality:

ADD/ADHD is one disorder that signals a deficit neurological system. Research suggests that 44% of individuals with ADD/ADHD will have one additional disorder, 30% will have two other disorders; and 11% will have an additional three disorders. Of these, 50-70% also have Oppositional Defiant Disorder and 30-40% have Conduct Disorders. Literature on language disorders suggest that at least 80% of learning disabilities are caused by language disorders, and most children with ADD/ADHD also exhibit learning disabilities. If a child is diagnosed with ADD/ADHD, it is important that a referral be made for speech-language testing, as well as other professional areas. Chapter 2 discusses other areas that can be at risk for children with ADD/ADHD.

Myth:

If ADD/ADHD is diagnosed, the child must be classified under "Special Education" in the school system.

"I don't want the school system to know she's ADD/ADHD. That means she'll have to be put in special classes."

Reality:

Not all children with ADD/ADHD meet criteria for special education enrollment, which requires an Individualized Educational Program (IEP). Many children with the disorder are accommodated under Section 504 of the 1973 Rehabilitation Act, which allows a list of recommendations within the regular education structure. Other children diagnosed with ADD/ADHD are able to manage their symptoms without special modifications in an academic setting. School personnel often receive inservice information on how to accommodate children with ADD/ADHD as part of their professional training and implement strategies as part of the normal classroom routine. Chapters 2 and 4 discuss legal provisions and requirements in conjunction with ADD/ADHD.

Myth:

There is a set intervention that works for children with ADD/ADHD.

"It's the teacher's fault that my child is still struggling in the classroom. She just doesn't know how to deal with ADD/ADHD."

Reality:

It is easy to place blame, but the fact is that there is no cookbook for dealing with ADD/ADHD. The disorder is evidenced individually and strategies and accommodations must always be adjusted and explored for each student. Understanding the neurology of learning and having experience with a diverse array of techniques is always helpful. Chapters 7, 8, and 9 present a wide variety of suggestions for intervention across the home and school settings.

Summary

With the re-authorization of IDEA, the defined role of the general educator has expanded and become more important. Children are increasingly placed in a least restrictive environment that requires that educational professionals function as a coordinated team. Everyone must have a vested interest in determining how to insure each student's success. Federal legislation has reinforced the reality of the general educator being faced with the dilemma of how to program for an increasingly diverse population. There are many more students with the characteristics of ADD/ADHD whose needs must be met.

The Source for ADD/ADHD was written with those challenges in mind. The realities introduced in this section will be developed in subsequent chapters to address the questions of those professionals who are responsible for designing and implementing educational programs for children with ADD/ADHD. Hopefully the material will also stimulate new thoughts to increase your confidence and success in intervening on ADD/ADHD.

Chapter 2

Definitions of ADD/ADHD

Case Example—Teacher's Perspective

Corey is a kindergarten student who is six years old. He displays both social and academic deficits in the school setting. He has a short attention span and can't sit still for longer than fifteen minutes. He's very impulsive, blurting out answers and comments without raising his hand or giving other students a chance to respond. His constant movement annoys other children in group time on the floor. He usually is picking at the student next to him, playing with the other's shoelaces, making faces and noises, or clowning around. It seems like he purposely answers wrong sometimes to make the other students laugh. He's disorganized and can't ever find his materials or get them together for art, P.E., or music. Motor coordination is poor and he is always falling and dropping things, which adds to the general chaos that seems to always surround him. Corey doesn't seem to apply himself consistently—sometimes showing perfect work and other times completely missing the directions and doing the entire worksheet incorrectly. He seems not to care when disciplined, shrugging off punishment or laughing. I have serious concerns about how to effectively focus and teach him in my classroom!

Medical Definition

What is Attention Deficit/Hyperactivity Disorder? ADD/ADHD is a syndrome disorder that is usually characterized by serious and persistent difficulty resulting in the following:

- poor attention span
- weak impulse control
- hyperactivity (not in all cases)

The characteristics usually onset during early childhood (before seven years of age), are chronic, and last at least six months. Individuals with ADD/ADHD usually experience difficulty with attention and learning, which can lead to subsequent problems in social skills, self-esteem, and behavior.

ADD/ADHD is a neurobiological disability that is estimated to affect approximately 3-10% of the population. Five percent of school-aged children and approximately 2-4% of adults have ADD/ADHD. In the United States, ADD/ADHD is one of the most common causes of referral in family practice, pediatric, neurology, and child psychiatry clinics (Biederman & Faraone, 1996). The disorder is usually present more often in boys than girls at about a 3:1 ratio.

Although individuals with ADD/ADHD can be very successful in life, without accurate identification and treatment, the disorder can have serious consequences, including failure in school, depression, conduct disorder, failed personal relationships, and substance abuse. Early identification and treatment increase a positive prognosis for productive long-term outcomes.

ADD/ADHD encompasses a variety of symptoms associated with it. There are also different venues for identification of the problem, with the two primary sites being a medical diagnosis and an educational diagnosis. This section will review the diagnostic criteria for diagnosing ADD/ADHD as well as differentiate it from other associated types of disorders.

The Diagnostic and Statistical Manual of Mental Disorders, Fourth Edition (2000) is the definitive source for medical diagnosis of ADD/ADHD. In the DSM-IV, published by the American Psychiatric Association, the disorder is identified as Attention Deficit Disorder (ADD); however, three types of ADD are delineated:
- predominantly inattentive
- predominantly impulsive
- combined

Diagnostic Criteria for ADD/ADHD

A. Either (1) or (2):
  (1) six (or more) of the following symptoms of inattention have persisted for at least six months to a degree that is maladaptive and inconsistent with developmental level:

  Inattention
  a. often fails to give close attention to details and makes careless mistakes in schoolwork, work, or other activities
  b. often has difficulty sustaining attention in tasks or play activities

    c.   often does not seem to listen when spoken to directly

    d.   often does not follow through on instructions and fails to finish schoolwork, chores, or duties in the workplace (not due to oppositional behavior or failure to understand instructions)

    e.   often has difficulty organizing tasks and activities

    f.   often avoids, dislikes, or is reluctant to engage in tasks that require sustained mental effort (such as schoolwork or homework)

    g.   often loses things necessary for tasks or activities (e.g., toys, school assignments, pencils, books, or tools)

    h.   is often easily distracted by extraneous stimuli

    i.   is often forgetful in daily activities

(2) six (or more) of the following symptoms of hyperactivity-impulsivity have persisted for at least six months to a degree that is maladaptive and inconsistent with developmental levels:

Hyperactivity

    a.   often fidgets with hands or feet or squirms in seat

    b.   often leaves seat in classroom or in other situations in which remaining seated is expected

    c.   often runs about or climbs excessively in situations in which it is inappropriate (in adolescents or adults, may be limited to subjective feelings of restlessness)

    d.   often has difficulty playing or engaging in leisure activities quietly

    e.   is often "on the go" or often acts as if "driven by a motor"

    f.   often talks excessively

Impulsivity

    g.   often blurts out answers before questions have been completed

    h.   often has difficulty awaiting turn

    i.   often interrupts or intrudes on others (e.g., butts into conversations or games)

B. Some hyperactive-impulsive or inattentive symptoms that caused impairment were present before age seven.

C. Some impairment from the symptoms is present in two or more settings (e.g., at school [or work] and at home).

D. There must be clear evidence of clinically significant impairment in social, academic, or occupational functioning.

E. The symptoms do not occur exclusively during the course of a Pervasive Developmental Disorder, Schizophrenia, or other Psychotic Disorder and are not better accounted for by another mental disorder (e.g., Mood Disorder, Anxiety Disorder, Dissociative Disorder, or a Personality Disorder).

When applying the DSM-IV criteria, the three primary subtypes could be summarized in the following list:

AD/HD primarily inattentive type (AD/HD-I):
- fails to give close attention to details and makes careless mistakes
- has difficulty sustaining attention
- does not appear to listen
- struggles to follow through on instructions
- has difficulty with organization
- avoids or dislikes tasks requiring sustained mental effort
- is easily distracted
- is forgetful in daily activities

AD/HD primarily hyperactive/impulsive type (AD/HD-HI):
- fidgets with hands or feet or squirms in chair
- has difficulty remaining seated
- runs about or climbs excessively
- acts as if driven by a motor
- talks excessively
- blurts out answers before questions have been completed
- difficulty waiting or taking turns
- interrupts or intrudes upon others

AD/HD combined type (AD/HD-C):
- individual meets both sets of attention and hyperactive criteria

The diagram on the following page illustrates ADD/ADHD and might help clarify the relationship among the three types.

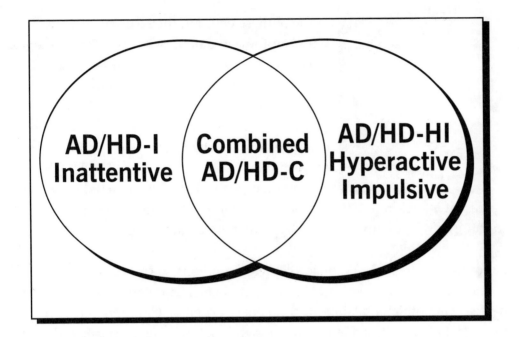

Associated Disorders with ADD/ADHD

Many of the symptoms associated with ADD/ADHD can also be symptoms of other problems, such as conduct disorders, depression, or anxiety. Due to the wide variety of disorders that can be mistaken for ADD/ADHD or that can co-exist with ADD/ADHD, it is always essential for a child to be carefully evaluated. "Look-alikes" might meet the diagnostic criteria for ADD/ADHD, but the symptoms could be present for different reasons. The diagnostic process must be careful and thorough so that treatment is focused and appropriate to the child's needs. Treatment strategies used may be quite different for a child with psychological problems rather than ADD/ADHD. Some of the psychomedical or medical disorders that can co-occur or mirror ADD/ADHD are described in the following section. Each will also be graphically represented to symbolize the relationship of the disorder with ADD/ADHD.

Depression

Depression is certainly common in children and adults. While it might seem contradictory to think of inattentive children with impulsive and hyperactive behaviors as depressed, the research suggests that 11% of individuals with ADD/ADHD are also depressed, although other sources indicate a range of 10-30%.

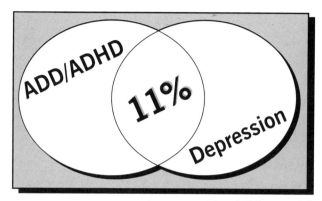

Some of these children may exhibit only passing symptoms of a depressed mood, but others persist in a pervasive mood disorder. The good news is that even though these children have ADD/ADHD symptoms, treatment for the depression can be quite successful. Researchers disagree as to whether depression occurs more frequently in children with ADD/ADHD than among their peers. However, when depression is present in children with an attention disorder, it is more likely to occur in children who do not have the hyperactivity component.

According to the DSM-IV, major depression involves physical symptoms, including changes in sleep patterns, eating habits, and energy levels. A decrease in both mental and physical energy occurs. Children may comment that no one likes them. Low motivation, lack of enthusiasm, reduced enjoyment of life, difficulty concentrating, slowed thinking, and indecisiveness can all be problems for the clinically depressed individual. A person who has depression may also exhibit memory problems and appear easily distracted, leading to the overlap or possible misdiagnosis with ADD/ADHD.

Anxiety Disorder

Anxiety Disorder occurs in approximately 11% of children who have ADD/ADHD, although research also suggests a range of 10-30%. There is also an overlap with depression. Of the children who are diagnosed with ADD/ADHD, 9% have both depression and anxiety disorders. (See graphic at the top of page 23.)

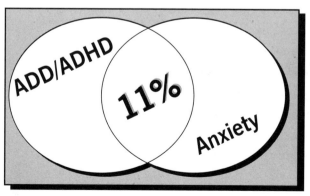

Some children can't seem to stop worrying. They feel on edge, have difficulty concentrating, are irritable, have muscle tension, or experience sleep disturbance. Even though many of the symptoms of an anxiety disorder may look the same as ADD/ADHD, the use of ADD/ADHD medication often worsens the symptoms of the anxiety disorder. The anxiety characteristics that a child displays can also mask the symptoms of ADD/ADHD, so that the ADD/ADHD remains undiagnosed. For an intelligent child whose ADD/ADHD is undiagnosed, the academic difficulties and underachievement can trigger high levels of anxiety, resulting in an initial diagnosis of panic or anxiety disorder, rather than ADD/ADHD. However, severe anxiety disorders, such as panic disorder and obsessive compulsive disorder, are rare in children with ADD/ADHD.

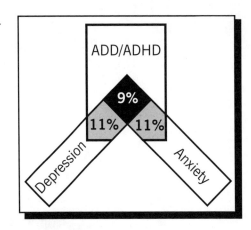

Bipolar Disorder

Another biomedical condition that can mimic ADD/ADHD is bipolar disorder. Bipolar disorder can present with impulsivity, inattention, hyperactivity, swings in high and low physical energy, along with behavioral and emotional ups and downs. It is sometimes difficult to tell ADD/ADHD and bipolar disorder apart because they share several common characteristics. The key difference seems to be that in ADD/ADHD, the symptoms, such as hyperactivity and poor

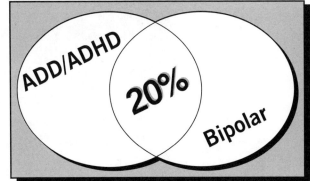

impulse control, are present consistently rather than evidenced in cycles. Research suggests that approximately 20% of individuals with ADD/ADHD may manifest bipolar disorder.

Dr. Barkley (1977) found that the majority of children with ADD/ADHD do not meet the criteria for bipolar disorder. An awareness of the symptoms of bipolar disorder may help avoid an incorrect diagnosis. The primary presenting symptoms of bipolar disorder are delineated below and on the following page:

1. Psychotic symptoms that reflect an impaired thought process, evidenced by gross distortions in reality. Rapid shifts from one thought to another can also occur. Children with ADD/ADHD may shift from one idea to the next, but they remain in touch with reality.

2. Severe temper tantrums that release a tremendous amount of physical and emotional energy. These tantrums generally last longer (30 minutes up to 2-4 hours) than for children who are not bipolar.

3. Pronounced irritability, especially in the morning.

4. Sleep disturbances, evidenced by difficulty sleeping through the night or severe nightmares with explicit terrifying images.

5. Aggression and destructiveness. Children with bipolar disorder may intentionally hit or hurt someone. In contrast, the misbehavior of a child with ADD/ADHD is often accidental.

6. Pronounced sexual awareness and interest, danger seeking, giddiness, and loud giggling. These characteristics can be observed as early as preschool years.

Oppositional Defiant Disorder/Conduct Disorder

In addition to the disorders mentioned previously, two other conditions occur frequently within ADD/ADHD—Oppositional Defiant Disorder (ODD) and Conduct Disorder (CD). Diagnostic criteria for both are defined within the DSM-IV. Children may begin to show signs of ODD/CD as early as six or seven years of age.

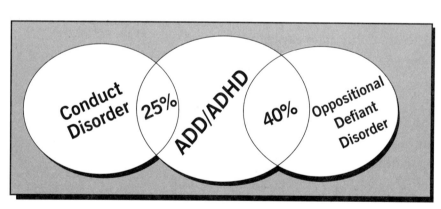

The Journal of American Academic Child & Adolescent Psychiatry (1996), reported that 5% of the total population demonstrates Oppositional Defiant Disorder. Within the ADD/ADHD population, 40% have ODD and 25% present with the more severe CD.

ODD describes children who are argumentative, hostile, defiant, and refuse to follow rules. For a diagnosis of ODD, four out of the eight behaviors listed on page 25 must be present, lasting for a period of at least six months.

- often loses temper
- often argues with adults
- often actively defies or refuses to comply with adults' requests or rules
- often deliberately annoys people
- often blames others for his or her mistakes or misbehavior
- is often touchy or easily annoyed by others
- is often angry and resentful
- is often spiteful or vindictive

Conduct Disorder describes children who have more serious behavior problems, such as persistent stealing, lying, destroying property, physical cruelty to animals or people, and fighting.

The diagnostic criteria for Conduct Disorder applies to children who have repeatedly violated the rights of other people. For a diagnosis, the child must manifest three or more of the following in the past 12 months, with at least one present in the past six months:

Aggression to people and animals:
- often bullies, threatens, or intimidates others
- often initiates physical fights
- has used a weapon that can cause serious physical harm to others (e.g., bat, brick, broken bottle, knife, gun)
- has been physically cruel to people
- has been physically cruel to animals
- has stolen while confronting a victim (e.g., mugging, purse snatching, extortion, armed robbery)
- has forced someone into sexual activity

Destruction of property:
- has deliberately engaged in fire-setting with the intention of causing serious damage
- has deliberately destroyed others' property (other than by fire-setting)

Deceitfulness or theft:
- has broken into someone else's home, building, or car
- often lies to obtain goods or favors or to avoid obligations (i.e., "cons" others)

- has stolen items of nontrivial value without confronting a victim (e.g., forgery, shoplifting)

Serious violation of rules:
- often stays out at night despite parental prohibitions, beginning before 13 years of age
- has run away from home overnight at least twice while living in parental or parental surrogate home (or once without returning for a lengthy period)
- is often truant from school, beginning before 13 years of age

Children with a combination of ADD/ADHD and Conduct Disorder have the most serious problems and the poorest prognosis. Individuals with Conduct Disorder are more likely to be expelled from school, break the law, abuse drugs, and be arrested.

Learning Disorder

The term *learning disabled* describes a neurobiological disorder in which a person's brain is structured or functions differently. These differences can interfere with the ability to think and remember information. A learning disability can negatively impact a person's ability to read, write, spell, listen, reason, recall, organize information, and perform math calculations. According to the National Institute of Health, 20% of the United States school population, or one in five Americans, are learning disabled.

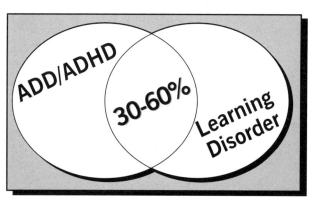

Individuals with ADD/ADHD frequently evidence difficulty learning in school. Research suggests that anywhere from 30-60% of children with ADD/ADHD also have a co-existing learning disorder. The DSM-IV differentiates Learning Disorders into Reading Disorder, Mathematics Disorder, Disorder of Written Expression, and Learning Disorder Not Otherwise Specified. This category will be further explored in the next section on Educational Definitions.

Communication Disorder

Children with ADD/ADHD are more likely to have a delayed onset of speech-language acquisition as compared to their peers (6-35% of ADD/ADHD, versus 2-6% of the general population). The typical language difficulties associated with ADD/ADHD include the following:

- pragmatic deficits—difficulty focusing on social cues so not able to monitor behavior adequately
- problem solving deficits—decreased focus can hinder recognition of important details necessary for basic problem solving
- auditory/language processing deficits—difficulty listening and attaching meaning to verbally presented information
- discourse deficits—difficulty managing topic maintenance, topic switch, and associative topic control in conversation

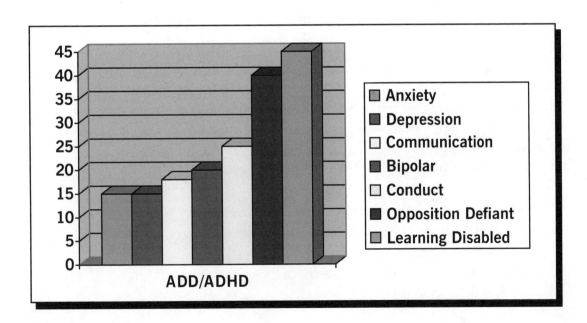

Below is a summary graph of the disorders commonly associated with ADD/ADHD. When a range has been provided for incidence, a middle point or average was used to chart the disorder. The chart illustrates that individuals with ADD/ADHD often experience additional problems as a result of the deficit.

The reported figures appear to be somewhat misleading. There is a dramatic discrepancy between the co-existence of a diagnosed communication/speech-language disorder (18%) and learning disability (45%). However, many students identified as learning disabled and ADD/ADHD receive services related to their academic deficits without referral to the speech-language pathologist. More appropriate services within a school setting should include a speech-language referral in addition to learning disabilities.

Educational Definition

Children with ADD/ADHD are covered by three federal statutes: the Individuals with Disabilities Education Act, Part B (IDEA); Section 504 of the Rehabilitation Act of 1973; and the Americans with Disabilities Act of 1990 (ADA). The U.S. Department of Education has the legal authority to interpret and enforce IDEA, and the Office of Civil Rights in the Department of Education interprets and enforces the provisions of Section 504 and ADA that pertain to education. These specific laws are explained in more detail later in this chapter. The Department of Education issued a Policy Clarification Memorandum in 1991 that defines a school's legal obligation to locate, identify, and evaluate children suspected of having ADD/ADHD (known as "child find"), and also to provide a free appropriate education and needed services for those who are eligible.

IDEA

Under IDEA, the federal government provides funding to the states so they can develop and maintain quality special education programs. To qualify for funds provided by this law, states must guarantee that students have a variety of services and rights available to them within the education system. These services include the following:
- Free and appropriate education (FAPE)
- Involvement of parents in educational decisions
- Nondiscriminatory evaluations and assessments
- An Individualized Educational Program (IEP)
- An education in the least restrictive environment (LEA)
- A right to due process

To be eligible under Part B of IDEA, "a child must be evaluated . . . as having one or more specified physical or mental impairments, and must be found to require special education and related services by reason of . . . these impairments." In other words, a diagnosis of ADD/ADHD is not enough to qualify a child for special education services—the ADD/ADHD must impair the child's ability to benefit from education.

The memorandum specifies that children with ADD/ADHD may be eligible for special education services under three categories defined by IDEA: other health impaired, specific learning disability, and seriously emotionally disturbed.

✔ *Eligibility for services under Other Health Impaired (OHI)*
The term "other health impaired" includes chronic or acute impairments that result in limited alertness, which adversely affects educational performance. Children with ADD/ADHD could be classified as eligible for services under "other health impaired" in instances where the ADD/ADHD is accompanied by chronic or acute health problems that impede sustained attention or focus, which adversely affects educational performance.

✔ *Specific Learning Disability*
Children with ADD/ADHD are more likely to have a learning disability, evidenced by difficulty acquiring academic knowledge in a classroom setting. Learning disabilities are generally most apparent in the basic psychological processes of understanding or using spoken or written language. These difficulties lead to weaknesses in reading, writing, spelling, and/or math skills.

Children with ADD/ADHD may qualify for special education in this category if they have coexisting specific learning disabilities; although, in some cases, ADD/ADHD alone may qualify a child to meet the criteria for this category. In defining specific learning disabilities, federal statutory language includes the term "minimal brain dysfunction," which is an earlier name for ADD/ADHD. Brain imaging studies underscore this category's continuing applicability and relevance for children with ADD/ADHD.

✔ *Seriously Emotionally Disturbed*
If a child is having serious behavior problems at school, personnel may label the student as demonstrating an emotional or behavioral disorder. Studies suggest that there is a high correlation between children receiving mental health services and ADD/ADHD. Within the educational system, this disability label can only be introduced when other major disabilities have been ruled out, which could account for the behavioral disruptions that interfere with learning.

To be eligible under this category, a child with ADD/ADHD must exhibit one or more of the following characteristics over a sustained period of time and to a degree that adversely affects educational performance:
- an unexplained inability to learn
- unsatisfactory personal relationships with teachers and peers
- inappropriate behavior and feelings
- general depression
- physical symptoms or fears resulting from personal or school problems

Section 504

Section 504 of the Rehabilitation Act is a civil rights law that prohibits discrimination against people with disabilities. Section 504 is aimed at eliminating discrimination by any program or activity that receives funding from the federal government. Under Section 504, a person with a disability is considered to be anyone with a physical or mental impairment that substantially limits one or more "life activities." Life activities include walking, breathing, speaking and/or hearing, seeing, learning, performing manual tasks, and caring for one's self.

Children may qualify for services to the handicapped under Section 504 of the Rehabilitation Act of 1973 if their ADD/ADHD substantially limits their ability to learn. Section 504 prohibits programs that receive federal dollars from discriminating against individuals with disabilities. It requires public schools to make accommodations for eligible handicapped children, whether or not they qualify for special education services under IDEA. Section 504 could, therefore, provide modifications for children with ADD/ADHD in regular classrooms, such as help with note-taking and changes in assignments and testing procedures.

ADA

The Americans with Disabilities Act prohibits discrimination against individuals with disabilities at work, at school, and in public accommodations, and is not limited (like Section 504) to those organizations and programs that receive federal funds. ADA requires schools to make reasonable accommodations for handicapped persons, and it applies to both public and private nonsectarian schools, from day care to graduate school.

Although the federal laws are similar in many ways, there are also some important differences.

1. Eligibility criteria for Section 504 is broader than for IDEA. Often children with ADD/ADHD who are unable to qualify for services under IDEA, can qualify under Section 504.

2. Services under IDEA are held to a higher standard than those under Section 504. Educational services under IDEA must be sufficient to allow a child to receive an educational benefit from his schooling. Under Section 504, educational services must be comparable to those received by students without disabilities. There is no requirement that the district insure educational benefit for the student within the services provided.

3. IDEA only covers students in the public school through grade 12; Section 504 covers students past high school to include enrollment in technical schools, colleges, and universities.

Discriminating the most appropriate method for insuring educational services to meet the needs of a child with ADD/ADHD can be a complex process, but a critical one. The input of a variety of professionals who function on an educational team is important to assist the family in the decision process.

Differentiating between the various educational options is developed in more detail in Chapter 4, which deals with diagnosis and referral procedures for appropriate intervention.

Questions & Answers

What can parents do to prevent a child with ADD/ADHD from also developing Oppositional Defiant Disorder (ODD) or Conduct Disorder (CD)?

One of the things parents should do is recognize that children with ADD/ADHD are at risk for becoming oppositional because of their emotional control problems. Consequently, parents need to start being regimented and structured in their parenting tasks when their child is at an early age. The key is to become proactive to prevent development of later problems.

One factor that helps predict which children might become oppositional is if the parent also has ADD/ADHD. If the parent is hyperactive, impulsive, emotional, or unregulated, the child lacks the rigorous controls necessary to prevent escalation into oppositional behavior.

Is ADD/ADHD going to keep my child from ever participating in activities such as driving a car, flying an airplane, or entering military service?

Having ADD/ADHD or taking medication in childhood in no way interferes with a child's ability to enter into the military, become a pilot, become a radio engineer, drive a car, or anything else he or she might want to become. But needing medication is an indicator that the disorder is severe enough to require management. This is something that may need to be discussed in conjunction with career options.

If, as a teacher, I suspect that a child suffers from ADD/ADHD, can I tell the parents it would be a good idea to seek a pediatric evaluation to look at the possibility of medication?

It is probably not a good idea to begin exploring the issue of a child's possible ADD/ADHD by telling the parents to have the child examined by a pediatrician for medication. The first step a teacher should take when a disability affects learning is a referral for possible identification and evaluation.

> *What are some aspects of ADD/ADHD that have*
> *the most impact on a prognosis?*

The following variables seem to influence the amount of improvement for future resolution of the problems associated with ADD/ADHD:

- IQ—the higher the better
- hyperactivity—less is better
- aggression—less is better
- age of detection/diagnosis—earlier is better
- socio-economic level—higher is better (improved access to services)

Chapter 3

Characteristics of ADD/ADHD

Case Example

"Seventeen professionals in two weeks haven't been able to figure out this kid who doesn't weigh forty pounds sopping wet and he sits there looking like he hasn't done a thing"(Woodward & Biondo, Living Around the Now Child, 1972). It's not getting any better. We've tried everything we can think of at home and nothing seems to work. The teachers report the same frustrations at school. They list all these behaviors and say that he is interfering with their ability to teach the rest of the class. He says he isn't doing anything wrong and is doing the best he can—but somehow he's always in trouble. He is such a puzzle. Just when I think I have him figured out, he responds differently than I ever expected. He's driving us all crazy—and we're driving him crazy! Someone needs to help us sort things out.

Observations of a Teacher

Behavioral characteristics of the child with ADD/ADHD place teachers in a quandary. Unfortunately, the child tends to present the ultimate challenge to professional competence. The result can become a mini-battlefield in the classroom, with the teacher determined to prevail over this little body placed in her charge. If the child becomes a threat to the teacher's control, confidence, sense of order and routine, or "normal" style of teaching, the child loses. It takes a confident, competent teacher to see the child and disorder label of ADD/ADHD as two separate entities. Teaching the child with ADD/ADHD should not become a power struggle between the child and the teacher. Both need to work together to overcome the neurological differences that constitute ADD/ADHD.

It is also important for the teacher to understand that ADD/ADHD is a performance problem in executing skills versus a learning disability, which is a processing problem (Goldstein & Goldstein, 1993). It isn't necessarily that the child's brain isn't capable of meaningfully handling the cognitive academic task; the problem is controlling the brain and body to attend to the stimulus presented so the brain has a chance to perform the processing.

Typical teacher comments reflect frustration, confusion, and exasperation with ADD/ADHD students. Ten example scenario quotes are provided, many extrapolated from *Living Around the Now Child* (Woodward & Biondo, 1972).

1. He can't sit still. He's on the go all the time. He's not mean or bad, just incredibly active.

2. She's smart and genuinely interested in a lot of things. She can talk about anything, but she can't seem to write a sentence or demonstrate her knowledge on a test or worksheet. Yet when she comes up to talk to me, she has all the right answers. Why can't she do it on her own?

3. He reacts to the slightest provocation. It doesn't take much to set him off. He's also physical with the other students. He grabs someone by the arm or pushes him or her to make a point, which causes trouble.

4. She makes me feel like a failure. I've been teaching for 15 years and I've never experienced anything like her. I've tried everything I know to try, and nothing works. When I was in school, they didn't say anything about working with students like her.

5. He is not working at his capacity. If I stand right next to him, he works fine, but as soon as I walk away he stops working. Or he works fast just to get it done, and then everything's wrong. If he would just apply himself and stay with it, he wouldn't have failing grades.

6. She's so messy and careless. Her desk is a cluttered mess, and she can't ever find anything. She loses things and isn't ever prepared. It's such a struggle to get her started.

7. I actually think he's pretty sensitive. If it looks like he's going to have trouble, he quits. When he gets something wrong, he's devastated and breaks down completely—either crying or screaming in anger. Sometimes I think he doesn't care, and other times I think he cares too much. Every time he makes a mistake, he apologizes, and I think he means it. But then he does it again. I'm at my wits end!

8. Every day I say, "It's going to be better. I'm not going to lose my temper or patience." On good days, I can make it to noon before I lose it. Most days I am climbing the walls within twenty minutes. Either he goes to another class, gets medicine, or I quit.

9. Sometimes I have to stop myself from laughing out loud at his antics. If he were the only child in my room, he would be such a joy. But I can't keep up with him and twenty-some other students. He requires so much special attention.

10. In spite of all the positive things about her, she is still the biggest problem I have in my class.

Observations of a Parent

Despite the incredible challenges that teachers face with children who have ADD/ADHD in an educational setting, the parents' problems are further magnified. A teacher only has to deal with the child for a relatively few hours per day in a controlled situation. Parents must cope with the unpredictable characteristics 24 hours a day, 7 days a week. Parents experience the behavioral characteristics with an increased intensity and frequency, as compared to the teacher.

Parents' reactions to the child with ADD/ADHD cover the continuum of emotions, from incredible guilt and blaming themselves, to totally giving up and blaming the child. In *Living Around the Now Child* (Woodward & Biondo, 1972), the following comments from parents were shared. They are organized into emotional reaction groups to provide a flavor for the turmoil the parents experience.

Frustration

- We've tried everything and nothing works.
- She doesn't seem to appreciate anything.
- He's on the move constantly and needs a lot of space.
- He never gets tired. He goes all day long and is up early in the morning ready to go.
- She says, "I'm sorry" and then turns around and does the same thing again!

Confusion

- He gets over things so quickly! I'm still angry and he's puckered up for a kiss of forgiveness and ready to move on.
- She has a high IQ but gets failing grades?!
- You can't ever predict what will set her off; it can be the least little thing.
- I don't understand. He can be so good, and then he can be *sooo* bad.
- Teachers say she doesn't try or apply herself. But at some things, she works till she drops or until it's just perfect.

Anxiety and Worry

- It's probably our fault, but we don't know what to do.
- If he's like this now, what will he be like when he's 18?
- She's so careless and impulsive; I worry about her safety.

- We feel like such failures as parents. Everyone blames us.
- School is such a negative experience. I just want him to be happy.

Helplessness

- I feel so sorry for her sometimes, I could just cry.
- Teachers say she doesn't care. Then why does she come home from school crying every day?
- He can be such an embarrassment when we go out in public.
- He thinks everyone is his friend, even when they're setting him up to get in trouble.
- Last night he prayed to be good.

Parents struggle to make sense of the enigma of ADD/ADHD and how it influences their child and affects their lives. ADD/ADHD can have a dramatic impact on parents. Goldstein (1993) summarized common effects of the disorder on parents as the following:
- increased stress
- greater psychopathology
- greater marital discord
- child exerts greater control

Professionals need to understand that the parents are not the cause of ADD/ADHD; the parents are also struggling to understand and cope with the disorder. Counseling, which includes concrete suggestions with functional application in the home environment, is welcomed by most parents. A tool that can be used to assess and identify specific sources of parent reactions is the *Parenting Stress Index* published by Psychological Corporation.

It is also important to listen carefully to parent comments. They provide valuable insight into the behavioral characteristic profile of a child with ADD/ADHD. The many facets of the disorder might not all be evidenced in the school setting. Parents can often fill in missing pieces of the ADD/ADHD puzzle.

Observations of a Child with ADD/ADHD

The primary reaction that children with ADD/ADHD must deal with is blame. They are constantly being scolded, punished, and lectured for being "different." Their "differences" are something they did not choose, and often, they cannot control. Yet the rest of the world often fails to realize the child's confusion and frustration with his own behavior. The "differences" do not stem from ulterior motives or a desire to be bad. These children are often coping the best way they can with a world that continually challenges and stretches their abilities to exist in harmony with others.

Research suggests that females with ADD/ADHD demonstrate some behavioral differences, including being more moody, emotional, and less aggressive than males. Perhaps the common trait is a tendency for children with ADD/ADHD to tell it like it is! Here are a few examples of quotes from children with ADD/ADHD.

- Why is everyone always mad at me?
- Sometimes I can do it, sometimes I can't.
- Everything seems so hard when I don't have help.
- I don't know why I did it.
- I don't like it when other people think I'm stupid.
- I can't ever find anything.
- They make me do stuff that's easy!
- I *have* to do it fast or I'll forget the answer.
- How long do I have to sit here?
- I wish I wasn't born. I'm nothing but trouble for Mom and Dad and my teachers.

Behavioral Characteristics

The child with ADD/ADHD *is* "different"! Behavior can seem unpredictable, random, and bizarre. It becomes a never-ending guessing game for parents and professionals to predict how the child will respond in situations. Most of all, the child is a source of frustration to himself and others.

There are multiple checklists and resources available that list and discuss characteristics of ADD/ADHD. Some of the lists are extensive, citing behaviors for pages and pages that simply overwhelm parents and professionals. Using various resources, we compiled a behavioral checklist for ADD/ADHD that categorizes presenting behaviors into eight major groups. Each listing below provides examples of behaviors that would be classified in that category. These behaviors have been converted to a screening checklist that is provided at the end of the chapter on pages 51-52.

Helplessness

- short attention span
- difficulty concentrating (especially on tasks that are routine and repetitive)
- difficulty listening
- difficulty starting and completing tasks
- difficulty following directions (especially with multiple steps)
- daydreams
- poor attention skills—selective, focused, sustained, divided

Impulsivity

- talks or acts without thinking
- difficulty waiting for turn
- rushes through assignments
- asks irrelevant questions
- calls out answers or questions in class
- outbursts
- shifts constantly from one task to next
- needs supervision
- doesn't think about consequences

Hyperactivity

- high activity level
- runs around constantly
- climbs on things excessively
- difficulty sitting still
- fidgets
- busy with physical activity unrelated to task
- loud or excessive verbalizations/vocalizations

- excessive movement in sleep
- always on the go; seems driven by a motor
- chatters incessantly

Disorganization

- forgets assignments and materials
- loses and misplaces things
- difficulty following sequential directions
- sloppy; messy
- poor sense of time

Social Skills Deficits

- immature and demanding; bossy
- easily frustrated; low tolerance
- overly sensitive
- emotionally over-reactive
- difficulty expressing feelings
- difficulty accepting responsibility for behavior
- frequent arguments or fights
- can't stand to lose; competitive
- blames difficulties on others
- plays with younger children

Difficulty Delaying Gratification

- rushes to finish work
- wants to be first
- can't wait for special occasions
- wants things NOW
- badgers, whines, nags

Emotional

- temper tantrums
- overly excited in groups
- not aware of what others are thinking
- broadcasts emotions to those around

- experiences feelings intensely
- demonstrates emotions in extreme exaggerated manner (e.g., silly, traumatic)

Noncompliance

- difficulty following rules
- ADD passively noncompliant; ADHD aggressively noncompliant
- strong willed; stubborn
- disregards dos and don'ts but can state them

Developmental Profile

Children with ADD/ADHD display different behavioral characteristics of the disorder as they progress from infancy to adulthood. Though not all children will exhibit all signs described in the stages represented, the following section explains what might be observed as a child develops through the life span with ADD/ADHD. A short narrative explanation is provided in the following section, followed by a summary chart of research studies documenting developmental characteristics.

- **Infancy**

  According to T. Phelan, Ph.D., the infant signs of ADD/ADHD are not as reliable as the behavioral characteristics described at later stages. However, there is a tendency for the "ADD/ADHD-to-be" infants to show more negative responses to new situations and to spend more time in negative moods. Children likely to develop ADD/ADHD can show overly intense emotional reactions, disturbed sleep patterns, and feeding difficulties during the very first year of development.

- **Toddlers**

  Many experts believe that it is possible to identify 60-70% of children with ADD/ADHD by two to three years of age. By this stage of development, noncompliance and stubbornness can already be extreme. If a child is the first born in a family, it might be difficult for the parents to discriminate if they are experiencing the "terrible twos," if a child is "all boy," or if a disability is showing early signs of onset. Once a child learns to walk, she might always be on the go.

Many of the children with ADD/ADHD are accident-prone and exhibit coordination difficulties. They often stop taking naps at an early age and become very demanding of attention, unable to play alone. Children with ADD/ADHD demand constant parental surveillance at this stage of development, as their high activity and insatiable appetite for stimulation requires an ever-watchful eye. If there are siblings, sibling rivalry can be extremely intense.

- **Preschool Ages: 3-5 Years**
  As the child with ADD/ADHD gets older, noncompliance in public situations can become more of an issue, often creating embarrassing situations for the parents. Peer problems begin to emerge as the child with ADD/ADHD moves from parallel play to more interactive play. Parents begin to experience phone calls from preschool programs and kindergarten teachers about the child's misbehavior. At this stage of development, it becomes apparent that typical discipline techniques don't work for children with ADD/ADHD. Methods of discipline, such as time-out, positive reinforcement, and punishment, are not effective with most of these children. Mounting frustration between adults and the child with ADD/ADHD can generate temper tantrums in the child that are totally out of proportion with the situation.

- **School Ages: 5-12 Years**
  Once the child with ADD/ADHD is enrolled in school, the structured demands to sit still and concentrate increase dramatically. School complaints become more frequent and often revolve around the child being described as "immature." Difficulties in learning begin to emerge, and the child with ADD/ADHD may be referred for a special education eligibility evaluation. Retention is often considered and recommended by classroom teachers. The child with ADD/ADHD may become more of a loner at this stage of development, with characteristics expanding to include defiant acting-out behaviors, such as lying, fighting, and stealing. The child's self-esteem can also begin to decline because of feeling inadequate or constantly being disciplined in the school setting.

- **Adolescence**

  By adolescence, most children with ADD/ADHD will begin to out-grow the gross-motor hyperactivity, although they may remain some-what fidgety at times. Peer problems can continue to escalate, or the children might begin to associate with friends who don't like school or are troublemakers. Teens sometimes test limits by becoming involved in anti-social acting out, such as truancy, vandalism, theft, or other problems in violation of the law. Adolescents with ADD/ADHD are also at greater risk for chemical abuse.

  Academically, the adolescent may be one to two years behind in cer-tain subjects due to her inability to pay attention. By this stage of development, the family feels a great sense of frustration with the child's behavior, especially with the frequent arguments at home about anything from school to chores. The child now runs a greater risk for depression and negativity regarding her life in general. There is also some evidence that children with ADD/ADHD are worse drivers than their peers without ADD/ADHD.

- **Adulthood**

  Since a child with ADD/ADHD cannot "outgrow" the disorder, adults with ADD/ADHD exist. The problems an adult with ADD/ADHD experiences are not outgrown but can moderate in severity and impact. Possible residual symptoms include inattention, impulsivity, and over-arousal. If these characteristics remain, they can hamper a person's job as well as personal relationships through-out the adult years. Emotional aspects of ADD/ADHD also need to be monitored. Depression and poor self-confidence can negatively impact general educational and economic achievement. The profes-sional level attained by individuals with ADD/ADHD is often less than one might expect based on innate ability. Adults with ADD/ADHD tend to move and change jobs frequently.

The table on the following pages summarizes the developmental course of ADD/ADHD using research studies to substantiate the profile.

Developmental Course of ADD/ADHD

	Study	Child Characteristics
Infancy	Campbell et al. (1982)	Excessive crying, drowsiness; colic, feeding problems; sleep disturbances
	Kaplan & Saddock (1985)	Undue sensitivity; aversive response to stimuli; sleep very little; cry a lot, irritable
	Knobel et al. (1959)	EEG abnormalities (occipital lobe)
	Waldrop et al. (1978)	Head and facial abnormalities
	Weiss & Hechtman (1986)	Difficult, impossible to soothe; excessive/little sleep; restless sleep, awake easily; unresponsive; colic, poor sucking; crying while eating; irregular eating; late in babbling; not cuddly; little smiling
	Wender (1987)	Temperamental differences; deficient neurotransmitters; siblings likely to be ADD; fathers likely to be ADD
	Werry et al. (1964)	Early mother-child difficulties due to excessive crying, colic & feeding problems
Toddlers	Battle & Lacy (1972)	Moms feel negative toward child, interact less frequently, less affectionate; infants were less compliant
	Mash & Johnston (1983)	Moms have high stress; moms have lower self-esteem (problems of child perceived worse with low esteem in mom); stress mother/child interaction
	Sroufe & Waters (1982)	Attachment ratings at age 12-18 months related to attending, focusing & social relatedness in preschool
Preschool	Barkley et al. (1985)	Parental stress at zenith when child is between 3-6 years
	Campbell et al. (1978)	Excessively active; noncompliant; difficult to toilet train
	Campbell et al. (1982)	Shift activities in free play; high activity levels during structured activities; impulsive responding
	Pelham & Bender (1982)	Rejected by peers
	Schleifer et al. (1975)	Hyperactive similar to normals in free play; true hyperactives (problems home and school) do less well than normals and situational hyperactive (problems home or school); parents of true hyperactives more frustration and stress than parents of normals or situational hyperactives; true hyperactives differ on motor impulsivity & field independence
	Campbell et al. (1977)	3-year follow-up on Schleifer (1975), children now 6-8 years; true hyperactives higher than situational on out-of-seat & off-task; true & situational hyperactives problems in elementary school, more disruptive, lower self-esteem than normals; hyperactive children had negative impact on classroom, teacher & other children
	Weiss & Hechtman (1986)	Number of referrals for hyperactivity increase for 3-4 year olds; environmental demands on child increase; negative encounters between child & others

Study	Child Characteristics
Early Childhood	
Barkley (1989)	Poor school performance; fail to finish assignments; disruptive in class; poor social relations; LD may become apparent
Campbell (1990)	Socialization is difficult; chaotic, punitive home makes socialization less likely; consistent, supportive, structured home helps some but not all ADHD children; symptoms change over time
Douglas (1983)	Primary deficits; attentional, inhibitory, arousal & reinforcement deficits; secondary deficits; low motivation, impaired metacognition, limited higher-order schemata (concepts & strategies)
Douglas & Peters (1979)	Extremely sensitive to presence/absence of reinforcers
Freibergs & Douglas (1969)	Learn at normal rates under 100% reinforcement schedule
Ross & Ross (1982)	Aggressive, oppositional behavior may appear; ADHD with aggression more severe problems later than ADHD children
Weiss & Hechtman (1986)	Most referrals grades 1-3; behavioral & cognitive disorders resemble syndrome; constellation of behaviors; behaviors impact on achievement; demands increase (structure); attention is low; environment is boring, repetitive, not reinforcing, not motivating; cycle of poor self-esteem & depression related to school performance
Wender (1987)	Low frustration tolerance; cycle of social difficulties, temperament & experience result in low self-esteem; may take risks, engage in dangerous acts to gain attention & enhance self image; family stress & sibling rivalry
Adolescence	
Barkley (1989)	Family conflicts centered on problems following rules & assuming responsibilities
Barkley et al. (1990)	After 8 years, 71% are ADHD; 59% Oppositional Defiant Disorder (DSM III-R); 43% Conduct Disorder (DSM III-R); 10% drop-outs; more likely to fail a grade; more likely to be expelled; divorce & separation higher
Blouin et al. (1978)	ADD vs. teens w/other school problems; ADD more conduct problems, impulsivity, hyperactivity, higher scores on self-injury scale & used more alcohol; behaviors normalized 16-21 years for majority (60%); 31% full syndrome symptoms; 9% still show difficulties; teens with symptoms; 48% antisocial; 10% substance abuse, same % as controls; early aggression in childhood predicts later antisocial (especially when mean, calculated and deliberate)
Mendelson et al. (1971)	13-year-olds identified between 8-10 years of age; 25% in special education; 2% in training schools; 2% in psychiatric hospitals; 70-80% restless & distractable; 26% history of antisocial problems; 17% juvenile court
Schachar et al. (1981)	Pervasive hyperactivity predicts persistent psychiatric disorders 9-14 years
Taylor (1986)	Pervasive hyperactivity predicts persistent psychiatric disorders & academic failure

	Study	Child Characteristics
Adolescence	Weiss & Hechtman (1986)	Original symptoms diminish replaced by antisocial, school & social problems; repeated antisocial behavior varies (10%, 25% to 45%) including serious crimes (assault with deadly weapon); primary social learning deficit combined with impaired parent/child relationship
	Wender (1987)	Do not experience pleasure normally (thrill seeking behaviors may be high); self-control problems; lack empathy & awareness of how they affect others; 50% outgrow symptoms; 25-30% symptoms diminish/others persist; 10-25% mixed, unclear outcome
Adult	Barkley (1989)	75% show depression; 23-45% juvenile convictions & adult antisocial disorders; 27% may be alcoholic
	Weiss et al. (1985)	15 year follow-up, self-esteem & social problems persist

Information taken from Teeter, P.A. "Attention-deficit hyperactivity disorders: A psychoeducational paradigm," *School Psychology Review, Vol. 20, No. 2,* 1991, pp. 266-280.

Impact of ADD/ADHD

The impact of ADD/ADHD can be pervasive, as delineated in the developmental section. The four primary areas that are affected are social, personal/psychological, physical, and learning. Each of these areas is illustrated in the diagram and described in the following section.

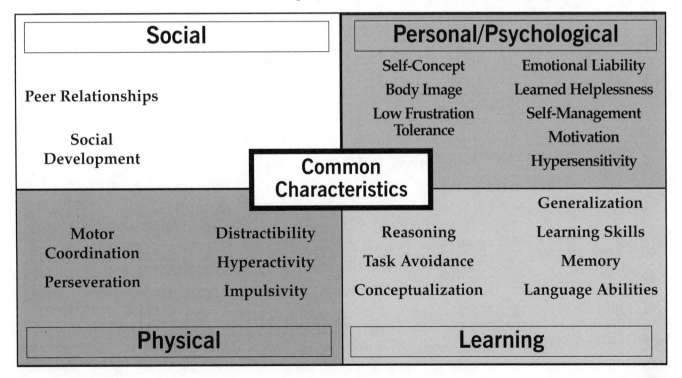

- **Social**

Social development is volatile as a result of the consequences of ADD/ADHD on other aspects of a child's life. The physical differences, psychological overtones, and learning difficulties play havoc with the ability to form meaningful friendships with peers and close relationships with siblings and other family members. Relatives may be intimidated or resistant to spending time with the child who has ADD/ADHD because of behavioral management issues. Friends' parents may hesitate to invite the child with ADD/ADHD to play dates, birthday parties, and other activities because of being overwhelmed by their exuberance. Peer relationships can suffer throughout life when people can't separate the ADD/ADHD disability symptoms from the individual who has them. Sometimes children with ADD/ADHD are never really given a chance by others. The disability characteristics interfere with the opportunity for peers to get to know them.

- **Personal/Psychological**

The emotional well-being of children can be significantly impacted by the presence of ADD/ADHD during their formative years. The constant negative comments regarding their behavior are likely to influence the development of personal feelings about themselves. Self-concept is more likely to be poor, reflected in a lack of confidence and an inaccurate idea of their own abilities and self-worth. Body image can also be affected, rarely viewing themselves as others see them. The ability to effectively manage themselves and their reactions can also be problematic, leading to emotional outbursts and mood swings. Children with ADD/ADHD can also be defensive, and always expecting the worst. This leads to low tolerance for criticism or suggestions and hypersensitivity to any comments that could be interpreted as critical. Other difficulties include learned helplessness—always relying on someone else to meet their needs, and poor self-motivation to push themselves to succeed unless a concrete, immediate reinforcement is offered for attaining a goal.

- **Physical**

ADD/ADHD is a neurological disability that significantly modifies a child's general physical status. The child cannot seem to sit still when the hyperactivity component is present, but cannot sustain attention to a task in either case. The physical differences can include distractibility, impulsive motor movements, perseverative verbal and motor actions as if the child's system is stuck, and motor coordination problems, making the child appear awkward or clumsy. Not all children within the ADD/ADHD profile will demonstrate problems in all areas mentioned. For example, some children demonstrate good motor coordination for athletic-type activities, but they lack the concentration to adequately apply their natural talents in the structure of team sport situations.

• **Learning**
Children with ADD/ADHD are at risk for a variety of learning problems in conjunction with the disorder. One major area is the development of general language skills. Language knowledge forms the foundation for academic learning. If language acquisition is delayed due to attention problems, academic learning is also likely to be negatively impacted. Being able to conceptualize ideas, reason through problems, and generalize knowledge acquired into other areas are learning skills impacted by the language deficits. Additional learning problems can include task avoidance, poor memory, and weak strategies for learning.

Questions & Answers

What can be done to help the adolescent and young adult with ADD/ADHD?

The first step is to identify and accept ADD/ADHD as a problem and the second is to learn about the disorder.

Counseling improves self-acceptance and understanding. Tutoring teaches the adolescent strategies for studying, learning, and organizational skills. As with the younger child with ADD/ADHD, environmental adaptations are necessary in the classroom. Adolescents and young adults should receive vocational counseling and be taught marketable skills for jobs that are tolerant of ADD/ADHD characteristics.

Medication is a treatment option that will be discussed in later chapters; however, it is important that an adolescent become comfortable with the reasons for medication. It used to be that children were taken off medication at puberty, but experts now suggest that it is beneficial for adolescents and adults to continue taking medication. There are many college students and adults on medication for ADD/ADHD to help with studies and job performance.

If children do not outgrow ADD/ADHD and will grow up to be adults with ADD/ADHD, what are the characteristics of adult ADD/ADHD?

Some of the characteristics of adult ADD/ADHD are listed below.
- chronic forgetfulness
- problems with time management, such as deciding how long a task will take and allotting appropriate time to the task
- tendency to take on too many tasks or projects than can be realistically managed
- generally disorganized lifestyle, e.g., chronically late, rushing, unprepared
- difficulty managing checkbook or finances
- frequent moves and job changes
- tendency to speak without considering the reaction
- tendency to interrupt others in conversation
- difficulty managing paperwork on the job
- difficulty controlling temper

How long have we known about ADD/ADHD as a disorder? Why does it seem to be diagnosed or present so frequently now?

ADD/ADHD characteristics have always been present in the population, but the disorder might not have carried so many penalties until more modern times. Children today face more demands when they start school. School experiences begin at a younger age and children are expected to show self-control and restraint earlier. They are expected to know how to conduct themselves and learn productively in group situations. Society has moved from an agricultural society with lots of outdoor movement and activity to more of an information/education-based society. What we are finding now is that there are groups of children who cannot meet these expectations as easily.

The Source for ADD/ADHD

ADD/ADHD Screening Checklist

Helplessness

- ❏ Short attention span
- ❏ Difficulty concentrating (especially on tasks that are routine and repetitive)
- ❏ Difficulty listening
- ❏ Difficulty starting and completing tasks
- ❏ Difficulty following directions (especially with multiple steps)
- ❏ Daydreams
- ❏ Poor attention skills—selective, focused, sustained, divided

Impulsivity

- ❏ Talks or acts without thinking
- ❏ Difficulty waiting for turn
- ❏ Rushes through assignments
- ❏ Asks irrelevant questions
- ❏ Calls out answers or questions in class
- ❏ Outbursts
- ❏ Shifts constantly from one task to next
- ❏ Needs supervision
- ❏ Doesn't think about consequences

Hyperactivity

- ❏ High activity level
- ❏ Runs around constantly
- ❏ Climbs on things excessively
- ❏ Difficulty sitting still
- ❏ Fidgets
- ❏ Busy with physical activity unrelated to task
- ❏ Loud or excessive verbalizations/vocalizations
- ❏ Excessive movement in sleep
- ❏ Always on the go; seems driven by a motor
- ❏ Chatters incessantly

Disorganization

- ❏ Forgets assignments and materials
- ❏ Loses and misplaces things
- ❏ Difficulty following sequential directions
- ❏ Sloppy; messy
- ❏ Poor sense of time

ADD/ADHD Screening Checklist, *continued*

Social Skills Deficits

- ❏ Immature and demanding; bossy
- ❏ Easily frustrated; low tolerance
- ❏ Overly sensitive
- ❏ Emotionally over-reactive
- ❏ Difficulty expressing feelings
- ❏ Difficulty accepting responsibility for behavior
- ❏ Frequent arguments or fights
- ❏ Can't stand to lose; competitive
- ❏ Blames difficulties on others
- ❏ Plays with younger children

Difficulty Delaying Gratification

- ❏ Rushes to finish work
- ❏ Wants to be first
- ❏ Can't wait for special occasions
- ❏ Wants things NOW
- ❏ Badgers, whines, nags

Emotional

- ❏ Temper tantrums
- ❏ Overly excited in groups
- ❏ Not aware of what others are thinking
- ❏ Broadcasts emotions to those around
- ❏ Experiences feelings intensely
- ❏ Demonstrates emotions in extreme exaggerated manner
  (e.g., silly, traumatic)

Noncompliance

- ❏ Difficulty following rules
- ❏ ADD passively noncompliant; ADHD aggressively noncompliant
- ❏ Strong-willed; stubborn
- ❏ Disregards dos and don'ts but can state them

Chapter 4

Diagnosis of ADD/ADHD

Case Example

Derek is repeating first grade. His teacher initiated a referral after discussing some of her concerns at a Parent-Teacher Conference. Derek is struggling in academic, social, and behavioral areas in the classroom setting. Most of the time he is happy and unconcerned about his behavior. He seems to understand the classroom expectations but doesn't abide by them. He cannot wait his turn. He interrupts the teacher and other students. He makes lots of noise and is constantly moving around and out of his desk. His feelings are easily hurt when reprimanded, yet he quickly forgets and does the same misbehavior twenty minutes later. He is disorganized, can't seem to concentrate, and never finishes assignments independently.

Preliminary assessment is a puzzle. Vision and hearing are fine. Academic performance is inconsistent, some days good with other days very poor. Reading, spelling, and math are falling significantly behind grade level performance. Derek seems to be attentive and understanding when group instruction and activities occur, yet individual worksheets and assignments do not reflect this perceived level of comprehension.

What is going on and what do we do with Derek?

Who Diagnoses ADD/ADHD?

A great deal of confusion exists in regard to who typically diagnoses ADD/ADHD. Determining if a child has ADD/ADHD is a multifaceted process. Biological and physiological problems can contribute to characteristics associated with the disorder. There is no single test to diagnose ADD/ADHD; therefore, a comprehensive evaluation is necessary to establish a diagnosis, rule out other causes, and determine the presence or absence of co-existing conditions.

There are several types of professionals who can diagnose ADD/ADHD, including school psychologists, private psychologists, psychiatrists, etc. In an educational setting, a multidisciplinary team evaluates a student to determine their unique needs within ADD/ADHD. Regardless of who does the evaluation, the use of the Diagnostic and Statistical Manual IV-TR (2000) criteria is necessary.

- **Medical Diagnosis**

   Within the medical community, pediatricians, physicians, neurologists, psychiatrists, and psychologists are all qualified to diagnose ADD/ADHD. Their roles begin to differentiate when you move into treatment options. Psychologists cannot prescribe medications, while the others can. Ongoing treatment and counseling for the child with ADD/ADHD are usually provided by psychiatrists and psychologists. A summary of these roles is provided in the following chart.

Role	Physician/ Pediatrician	Neurologist	Psychiatrist	Psychologist
Diagnose ADD/ADHD	Yes	Yes	Yes	Yes
Prescribe Medication	Yes	Yes	Yes	No
Provide Counseling	No	No	Yes	Yes

- **Educational Diagnosis**

   As presented in the Case Summary, when a teacher and/or parent thinks that a child is experiencing difficulty learning, federal laws (Section 504 and Individuals with Disabilities Education Act—IDEA) are in place to insure that schools evaluate children's unique educational needs. This is accomplished using a multidisciplinary team that includes a teacher and a specialist in the area of the suspected disability.

   Once a concerned party initiates a request to meet and discuss a child's difficulties in the school setting, a team meeting is convened. This step is often termed a pre-referral meeting. The initial team meeting may or may not include the parent; however, a variety of professionals in the school setting would meet to discuss characteristics of concern. Various districts title this group meeting differently, such as Teacher Collaboration Team, Teacher Assistance Team, Student Assistance Team Meeting, etc. Their purpose is to determine if more formal procedures are necessary to meet the student's needs. Information available is reviewed and a determination is made as to whether more extensive accommodations for the student are necessary.

The following flow chart summarizes the referral process and is further explained in the following section.

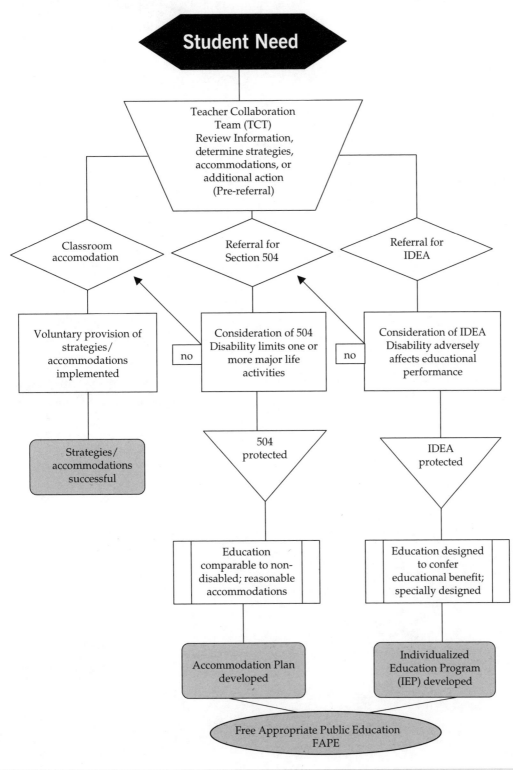

Flow Chart Explanation

- Many students with ADD/ADHD progress through the educational system with no difficulty or minimal problems. However, if a student begins to experience problems in the educational setting, that student's needs should be taken seriously and given appropriate consideration.

Student Need

- When a student begins to encounter difficulty in the educational setting, there is generally a collaborative team of teachers and adjunct professionals who meet to discuss specific concerns. That group functions in a sort of pre-referral process, by which educational personnel can determine if simple strategies or accommodations can be implemented in the classroom to resolve the problem, or if more formal modifications are necessary.

Teacher Collaboration Team (TCT) Review Information, determine strategies, accommodations, or additional action (Pre-referral)

- The decision that the collaborative team makes would be to address the student's needs in one of three ways: the classroom teacher could implement some modifications or accommodations that adequately address the concerns; the team could consider implementation of Section 504 to insure that limitations the student might be experiencing are addressed; or the team could decide to implement a full case study to meet the student's needs under IDEA.

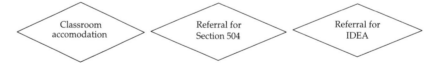

Classroom accomodation | Referral for Section 504 | Referral for IDEA

- If voluntary accommodations are successful to meet the student's needs, then the first column of voluntary strategies is completed.

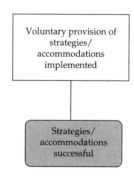

Voluntary provision of strategies/ accommodations implemented

Strategies/ accommodations successful

- If Section 504 is investigated, then the team meets to determine how modifications will be insured to provide reasonable accommodations for the student's needs. An accommodation plan is developed and filed to insure compliance with the suggestions since the student's right to modifications are protected by Section 504.

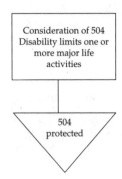

- If IDEA is initiated, then a full case study is performed to evaluate possible areas of student needs. A multidisciplinary staffing is convened to design an Individualized Education Program to meet the student's special needs. The right to the plan is protected under federal legislation.

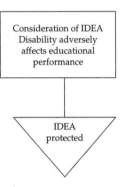

- At any point, the team could decide the more restrictive requirements are not necessary and move the procedure to the less restrictive accommodation model.

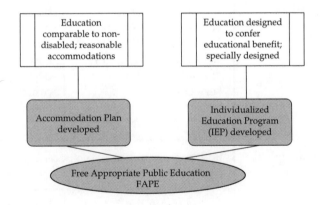

Collaborative Strategy Options

Component	Teacher Collaboration Team (TCT)	Section 504	IDEA
Purpose	A voluntary process that enables people with various expertise to generate solutions to mutually defined student problems.	A civil rights law that protects the rights of individuals with disabilities.	A federal statute whose purpose is to provide financial resources to states in their efforts to provide services to school-aged children with disabilities.
Responsibility to provide a Free and Appropriate Public Education (FAPE)	No requirement; Districts implementing TCT generally have developed a process and procedures.	Requires a written plan.	Requires a written Individual Education Program (IEP).
Special Education vs. Regular Education	A major outcome of TCT is to provide effective programming for students with diverse learning styles within a regular education setting.	A student is eligible as long as he meets the definition of a person with a disability, i.e., "has a physical or mental impairment which substantially limits a major life activity." The student does NOT require special education services.	A student can receive special education services if the multidisciplinary team determines that the student is eligible under one or more of the IDEA specific qualifying conditions and requires specially-designed instruction to confer educational benefit.
Procedural Safeguards	No requirement.	Both require notice to the parent/guardian with respect to identification, evaluation, and/or services.	
		Does not require written notice or consent.	Requires written notice and consent.

Component	Teacher Collaboration Team (TCT)	Section 504	IDEA
Evaluation	No requirement; Districts implementing TCTs generally have developed processes and procedures that include collection of relevant data from various sources in regard to the student.	Evaluation draws on information from a variety of sources in the area of concern. Decisions are made by a group knowledgable about the student.	A comprehensive evaluation assessing all areas related to the suspected disability. The child is evaluated by a multidisciplinary team.
Re-evaluation	No requirement.	Requires periodic re-evaluation.	Requires re-evaluations to be conducted at least every three years.
Due Process	No specific requirement for schools.	Both require districts to provide impartial hearing for parents who disagree with the identification, evaluation, or services provided.	
		Requires opportunity for parent participation. Details left to the discretion of local school district.	Federal law delineates specific requirements.

Federal Law Provisions for Education Services—
Section 504 versus IDEA

Section 504 of the Rehabilitation Act of 1973

✔ Provides appropriate education for children who do not fall within the disability categories specified in IDEA, Part B. Examples of potential conditions not typically covered under IDEA are communicable diseases (HIV, tuberculosis) medical conditions (asthma, allergies, diabetes, heart disease), temporary medical conditions due to illness or accident, and drug/alcohol addiction.

✔ Requires that a free appropriate public education be provided to each qualified child who is disabled, but does not require special education and related services under IDEA, Part B. A free appropriate education (FAPE) under Section 504 includes regular or special education and related aids and services that are designed to meet the individual student's needs and are based on adherence to the regulatory requirements.

The Source for ADD/ADHD 59

✔ Guarantees parents the right to contest the outcome of an evaluation if a local district determines that a child is not disabled under Section 504.

✔ Requires the local district to make an individual determination of the child's educational needs for regular or special education, or related aids and services, if the child is found eligible under Section 504.

✔ Requires the implementation of a written plan outlining accommodations to meet student needs.

✔ Requires that the child's education must be provided in the regular education classroom unless it is demonstrated that education in the regular environment with the use of supplementary aids and services cannot be achieved satisfactorily.

✔ Requires that necessary adjustments be made in the regular classroom for children who qualify under Section 504.

Individuals with Disabilities Education Act Part B, IDEA

✔ Requires that state and local districts make a free appropriate public education (FAPE) available to all eligible children.

✔ Requires that the rights and protections of IDEA are extended to children with ADD/ADHD and their parents.

✔ Requires that an evaluation be completed within 60 school days to determine if the child has one or more specified disabling conditions and requires special education and related services.

✔ Requires that children with ADD/ADHD be classified as eligible for services under the "Other Health Impaired" category in instances where ADD/ADHD is a chronic or acute health problem that results in limited alertness that adversely affects a child's educational performance. Children with ADD/ADHD can also be served under the categories of "Learning Disabilities" or "Seriously Emotionally Disturbed," if the evaluation finds these conditions are also present.

✔ Does not allow local districts to refuse to evaluate the possible need for special education and related services of a child with a prior medical diagnosis of ADD/ADHD solely by reason of that medical diagnosis. On the other hand, a medical diagnosis of ADD/ADHD does not automatically make a child eligible for services under IDEA.

✔ Requires that a full and individual evaluation of the child's educational needs must be conducted in accordance with requirements in IDEA. These requirements include that a multidisciplinary team must perform the evaluation and at least one teacher or other specialist with knowledge in the area of ADD/ADHD must be on the team.

✔ Requires that a due process hearing take place, at the request of the parents or school district, if there is disagreement between the local district and the parents over the request for evaluation, the evaluation, or the determinations for services.

IDEA Eligibility Categories Associated with ADD/ADHD

Children with disabilities as defined by PL 105-17 (IDEA '97) include mental retardation, hearing impairment (including deafness), speech or language impairments, visual impairments (including blindness), serious emotional disturbance, orthopedic impairments, autism, traumatic brain injury, other health impairment, or specific learning disabilities. Children aged 3-9 may be labeled as developmentally delayed. IDEA, therefore, includes ten disability categories plus developmentally delayed.

All children with ADD/ADHD are not automatically eligible under IDEA to receive special education and related services. To be eligible under IDEA, a child with ADD/ADHD must meet a two-pronged test of eligibility:

1) have a condition that meets one of the disability categories listed in IDEA; and

2) need special education and related services because of that disability.

Any of the ten categories can be applied to children with ADD/ADHD if they meet definition qualifications; however, most of the children with ADD/ADHD who qualify for special education services using the two-pronged test are typically categorized as being eligible under labels of Other Health Impaired, Learning Disabled, or Emotional Disturbance.

In September 1991, the Department of Education issued a memorandum entitled "Clarification of Policy to Address the Needs of Children with ADD/ADHD within General and/or Special Education, which was intended to clarify state and local responsibility under federal law for meeting the needs of children with ADD/ADHD in the educational system. Consistent with the 1991 memorandum, IDEA '97 further explained eligible conditions under "OHI" to include ADD/ADHD. Including ADD/ADHD as potentially eligible conditions under the IDEA does not add a new category label. It simply codifies the Department's long-standing policy related to serving these children.

- **Other Health Impaired**

  A student with a diagnosis of ADD/ADHD may be eligible for special education and related services under the category of Other Health Impaired. This determination must be made on a case by case basis. There are no state criteria specifically established for "Health Impairment." School districts must determine locally the criteria to be applied when determining a student eligible under this category. In making the determination the district must utilize the federal definition of OHI, which includes the following:

  > "...having limited strength, vitality or alertness, including a heightened alertness to environmental stimuli, that results in limited alertness with respect to the educational environment, that is due to chronic or acute health problems such as asthma, attention deficit disorder or attention deficit hyperactivity disorder, diabetes, epilepsy, a heart condition, hemophilia, lead poisoning, leukemia, nephritis, rheumatic fever, and sickle cell anemia; and adversely affects a child's' educational performance."

- **Learning Disability (LD)**

  The regulations for Public Law (P.L.) 105-17 and the Individuals with Disabilities Education Act (IDEA '97) define a learning disability as a "disorder in one or more of the basic psychological processes involved in understanding or in using spoken or written language, which may manifest itself in an imperfect ability to listen, think, speak, read, write, spell, or to do mathematical calculations."

  The Federal definition further states that learning disabilities include "such conditions as perceptual disabilities, brain injury, minimal brain dysfunction, dyslexia, and developmental aphasia." According to the law, learning disabilities do not include learning problems that are primarily the result of visual, hearing, or motor disabilities; mental retardation; or environmental, cultural, or economic disadvantage. Definitions of learning disabilities also vary among states.

  LD is a disorder that affects people's ability to either interpret what they see and hear or to link information from different parts of the brain. "These limitations can show up in many ways, such as specific difficulties with spoken and written language, coordination, self control, or attention. Such difficulties extend to schoolwork and can impede learning to read, write, or do math." (NIMH, 1990)

A complete definition of learning disabilities developed by the National Joint Committee on Learning Disabilities (NJCLD) appears as follows:

> Learning disabilities is a generic term that refers to a heterogeneous group of disorders manifested by significant difficulties in the acquisition and use of learning, speaking, reading, writing, reasoning, or mathematical abilities. These disorders are intrinsic to the individual, presumed to be due to central nervous system dysfunction, and may occur across the life span. Problems in self-regulatory behaviors, social perception, and social interaction may exist with learning disabilities, but do not by themselves constitute a learning disability. Although learning disabilities may occur concomitantly with other handicapping conditions (for example, sensory impairment, mental retardation, serious emotional disturbance), or with extrinsic influences (such as cultural differences, inappropriate or insufficient instruction), they are not the result of those influences or conditions. (1990)

The National Institutes of Mental Health (NIMH) describes learning disabilities as follows:

> Learning Disabilities (LD) is a disorder that affects people's ability to either interpret what they see and hear or to link information from different parts of the brain. These limitations can show up in many ways—as specific difficulties with spoken and written language, coordination, self-control, or attention. Such difficulties extend to schoolwork and can impede learning to read or write, or to do math.

- **Emotional Disturbances**

  Many terms are used to describe emotional, behavioral, or mental disorders. Currently, students with such disorders are categorized as having a serious emotional disturbance, which is defined under the IDEA as follows:

  > "...a condition exhibiting one or more of the following characteristics over a long period of time and to a marked degree that adversely affects educational performance:
  > (A) An inability to learn that cannot be explained by intellectual, sensory, or health factors;
  > (B) An inability to build or maintain satisfactory interpersonal relationships with peers and teachers;
  > (C) Inappropriate types of behavior or feelings under normal circumstances;
  > (D) A general pervasive mood of unhappiness or depression;
  > (E) A tendency to develop physical symptoms or fears associated with personal or school problems." [Code of Federal Regulations, Title 34, Section 300.7(b)(9)]

As defined by the IDEA, serious emotional disturbance includes schizophrenia but does not apply to children who are socially maladjusted, unless they have a serious emotional disturbance.

Balance of Professionals in Diagnosis

It is important that all individuals involved in diagnosis and intervention with children who have ADD/ADHD seriously evaluate their current models for provision of services. People would be appalled if they were forced to use the hairstyles, clothing, cars, televisions, etc. from the 1950s. Those models and styles are outdated and not reflective of how things are done today. Meeting the needs of students with special needs also requires some updating in procedures and styles. The method for doing business today is different. A model to illustrate this concept is provided below.

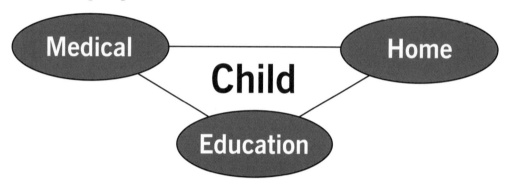

The child with ADD/ADHD must serve as the center of the system to balance all the other components. Diagnosis and intervention cannot occur effectively in isolation; all aspects—medical, home, education—must work in concert together. Each provides a focus, but at the same time, each must be flexible in working with and integrating the other components.

For example, medication in isolation is not the answer. Medical involvement might be necessary for a child to accomplish a productive state in the learning environment. However, teacher input is necessary to monitor positive and negative effects, resulting in modifications by the medical area.

The school setting also needs to make accommodations. Teacher modifications are always necessary for children with ADD/ADHD. However, it is important that the teacher not expect parents in the home setting to provide discipline and student strategies that will remediate behavior in the education setting. Parent discipline, structure, and consistency in the home by itself is not enough.

No one aspect can stand alone to "fix" ADD/ADHD. There must be balance in intervention for it to be effective. The status quo models don't hold up today. It is not how a teacher is structuring her classroom, how parents discipline in the home, or how doctors approach ADD/ADHD treatment. All three parts must work together to effectively balance the child in the center. Flexibility, awareness, and communication are all critical to successful diagnosis and planning to intervene on ADD/ADHD.

According to Goldstein & Goldstein (1993) there are eight types of data necessary for a thorough evaluation/diagnosis of ADD/ADHD:

1. History—behavioral, developmental and medical
2. Intelligence—an estimate of the child's level of reasoning, judgement, and thinking skills
3. Personality and Emotional Functioning—an overview of the child's self-esteem and emotional adjustment
4. Academic Achievement—an estimate of child's achievement in the school setting
5. Friends—an overview of the child's social perception, problem, and conflict resolution skills as well as social network
6. Parenting Skills and Discipline—an overview of the parents' perception of the problem as well as the strategies they use for intervention
7. School Behavior—teacher observation of the child's functioning within the school setting
8. Medical Evaluation—primarily to rule out the possibility that other medical problems exist

A variety of rating scales have been developed to determine the severity of problems associated with ADD/ADHD. These scales can offer valid and reliable information about a child, thus providing a means by which to compare a child's behavior to that of others of the same gender and age. Separate scales have been developed for parents and teachers since each informant will rate behaviors in their areas of involvement with the child.

Some of the more popular rating scales are:
- *Conners Teacher Rating Scale*
- *Conners Parent Rating Scale*
- *ADD-H: Comprehensive Teacher Rating Scale (ACTeRS)*
- *ADHD Rating Scale (Parents and Teachers)*
- *The School Situations Questionnaire*
- *The Home Situations Questionnaire*
- *The ADHD Rating Scale*

Questions and Answers

Does there need to be a diagnosis from a medical doctor in order to identify a child with ADD/ADHD as disabled under Section 504 or IDEA?

No. Schools are sometimes reluctant to qualify a child with ADD/ADHD unless they have a medical diagnosis that supports that eligibility; however, the federal regulations include no requirement that a district must have a medical evaluation in order to determine if a child is eligible for special modifications or educational services under Section 504 or IDEA. That does not mean that districts should ignore medical diagnoses when they are available. The district's obligation is to carefully consider all evaluation data.

What is a "Multidisciplinary" approach?

"Multidisciplinary" is a strategy in which different disciplines work together to identify a child's strengths and weaknesses in order to design educational and behavioral goals, to implement plans, and to follow up on the child's progress. A multidisciplinary team for a child with ADD/ADHD might consist of the physician, mental health professionals, learning disability specialist, speech-language pathologist, teachers, other educators, parents, and the child.

Is ADD/ADHD always a 504 Disability?

Not necessarily. The presence of ADD/ADHD must be judged to be "substantially limiting" to learning in order to qualify a child under Section 504. This determination is made by a group of education-based professionals who are knowledgeable about the child.

Is ADD/ADHD an educational disability under IDEA (Part B)?

ADD/ADHD does not stand alone as an education disability category under IDEA. Many children eligible for special education services under IDEA exhibit ADD/ADHD characteristics, but their special education eligibility labels are defined typically under categories of Other Health Impairment (OHI), Learning Disability (LD), or Emotional Disturbance (ED). However, other eligibility labels can be used if appropriate, such as Speech-Language Impairment (SLI).

Can a student with ADD/ADHD be placed in a special instructional program?

Yes, depending on the findings of the multidisciplinary staffing team. If, after a comprehensive educational evaluation, a child with ADD/ADHD meets existing disability category criteria and requires special education, then the student can be placed in special education services and/or classroom programs.

Chapter 5

Neurology of Learning Within ADD/ADHD

Case Example

Payton has a short attention span, is easily distracted, and his body is in constant motion. He is capable of working at grade level, but actual work performance is variable. Coordination is poor and his writing is jerky, sloppy, and has lots of erasures. He has great difficulty sequencing and cannot seem to follow directions. When asked a question, he never has an answer ready. Instead, he goes through an elaborate ritual of squeezing his eyes closed, hitting his hand against his forehead, grimacing in a frown, and repeating the question over and over again. All the theatrics seem to distract him further and cause other students to lose patience or laugh. He cannot sit still and is always coming up with an excuse for being out of his seat, such as needing a drink, sharpening his pencil, getting a paper, putting something away in his backpack, etc. It's no wonder Payton is having trouble learning—he spends all his time distracting himself and others!

The Neurology of ADD/ADHD

It is easy to put students' poor learning problems in the category of behavior. We can absolve ourselves of guilt by saying that the child doesn't care, doesn't want to learn, etc., but educators need to begin understanding the underlying mechanisms that govern teaching and learning. Focusing solely on behavioral issues can lead us to only a partial diagnosis and treatment of many complex learning behaviors associated with ADD/ADHD. The neurological system plays a critical role in how a student reacts and comprehends material presented in a classroom.

Behavioral observations do not necessarily imply voluntary chosen responses. Behaviors actually tell you how the neurological system is functioning and whether certain aspects are intact or impaired. The body's responses give us a window on what is going on inside the brain. The external manifestation (behavior) provides information on the internal workings.

Research is beginning to make gains in better understanding the neurological connection to the characteristics associated with ADD/ADHD. Some of the research impressions are summarized in the following sections.

Current Research Impressions on ADD/ADHD

- **Biology/Physiology**
Millions of parents trust that the professionals who teach their children know something about the brain and processes of learning. Most schools of education offer psychology, not neurology, courses. And these psychology courses, at best, provide indirect information about how children learn. Inservice training is directed toward

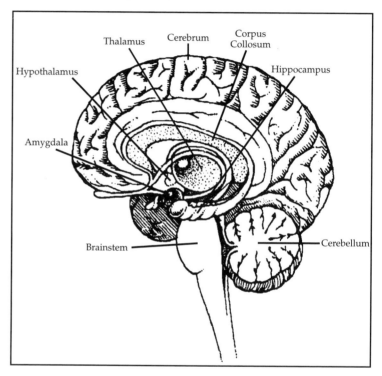

symptoms of problems, not a working knowledge of the brain. Questions about the brain remain, but we know enough to help educators develop effective teaching strategies. By understanding how the brain learns, we will improve our success working with children who have ADD/ADHD and other disorders.

The adult human brain weighs about three pounds. From the outside, the brain's most distinguishing features are its convolutions, or folds. These wrinkles are part of the *cerebral cortex* (Latin for "bark" or "rind"). We have two cerebral hemispheres, the left and the right. They are connected by bundles of nerve fibers, the largest known as the *corpus callosum*. The corpus callosum has about 250 million nerve fibers. Each side of the brain processes things differently. The original work of Nobel Prize Laureate Dr. Roger Sperry, who discovered the functioning differences between left and right brain hemispheres, remains valid; however, research has confirmed that both sides of the brain are involved in nearly every human activity. It's all a matter of timing and degree of involvement. What we can safely say about each hemisphere is that the left side processes "parts" (sequentially) and the right side processes "wholes" (gestalt).

To say that one side of the brain is logical or one side is creative is wrong because people can become very creative by following and using logical options, patterns, variations, and sequences. Both parts and wholes are important to learning. Neither should be emphasized at the expense of the other. Some of those who are promoting "right-brain thinking" might do more good by promoting "whole-brain thinking." Learners should be provided with global overviews that alternate between the "big picture" and the details. Good teaching needs to validate that we are "whole-brain learners."

Research using MRI and EEG scans headed by Dr. Paula Tallal, co-director of the Center for Molecular and Behavioral Neuroscience at Rutgers University, proved that the left hemisphere processes information faster than the right. Disorders can be dealt with more effectively by using new technology. For example, many learners who are labeled as "slow" may actually have a "slow" left hemisphere but shouldn't be labeled as disordered. These children are capable of learning in other ways. It is important to find specialists who can assist learners more effectively through an understanding of the neurology involved, rather than the resulting behavioral symptoms.

There are two kinds of brain cells—*neurons* and *glia*. While the majority of brain cells (90 percent) are glia, it is the remaining 10 percent, the neurons, that make the brain a thinking and learning organ. Though the brain contains fewer neurons than glia cells, they are essential to performing the brain's work.

A neuron consists of a *compact cell body*, *dendrites*, and *axons*. Neurons are responsible for information processing, and converting chemical and electrical signals back and forth. Two things are critical about a neuron when compared with other cells in the body. First, new research at Salk Institute in La Jolla, California, reveals that some areas of the brain can and do grow new neurons (Kempermann, Kuhg, and Gage, 1997). Second, a normal functioning neuron is continuously firing, integrating, and generating information; it's a virtual hotbed of activity.

About the thickness of your middle finger and coming up from the spinal cord is the *brain stem* area. It monitors and presents the physical world. It is instinctive, fast-acting, and survival-oriented. Researchers say it's the part of the brain that's responsible for learner behaviors such as:

- ✔ *social conformity*—common hairstyles, clothes, etc.
- ✔ *territoriality*—defending "my stuff, my desk, my room"
- ✔ *mating rituals*—flirting, touching, attracting another
- ✔ *deception*—often forms of subverted aggression
- ✔ *ritualistic display*—trying to get the social attention of peers
- ✔ *hierarchies*—the dominance of leaders, "top dog" behaviors
- ✔ *social rituals*—the repetitive & predictable daily behaviors

The territory in the middle of the brain includes the *hippocampus, thalamus, hypothalamus,* and *amygdala.* This *mid-brain* area represents 20 percent of the brain by volume and is responsible for the following:

- ✔ attention and sleep
- ✔ social bonding and attachments from parental bonding
- ✔ our hormones, feelings of sexuality
- ✔ sense of space and location
- ✔ our emotions, both positive and negative
- ✔ what is true, valid, and what we feel strongly about
- ✔ the formation of memories
- ✔ immediate expressiveness
- ✔ long-term memory

The *cerebrum* and the *neocortex* are the bulk of the brain. These areas used to be called our "thinking cap," but much more than thinking occurs here. The cerebrum and cortex includes the *frontal, occipital, parietal,* and *temporal* lobes and provides us with the following:

- ✔ thinking, reflection, consciousness
- ✔ some processing of emotions
- ✔ problem solving, computations
- ✔ language, writing, and drawing
- ✔ long-range planning, forecasting
- ✔ visualizing, envisioning
- ✔ reading, translating, and composing
- ✔ creativity in art, music, and theater

Each of the three areas of the brain influences the other.

The brain is energy inefficient. It is about 2 percent of the body's adult weight, but it consumes about 20 percent of the body's energy. How does the brain get its energy to learn? Its primary source is blood, which supplies nutrients like glucose, protein, trace elements, and oxygen. The brain gets about 8 gallons of blood each hour and about 198 gallons per day. In addition, water provides the electrolytic balance for proper functioning. The brain needs 8 to 12 glasses of water a day for optimal functioning. Dehydration is a common problem in school classrooms, leading to lethargy and impaired learning (Hannaford, 1995). A child shouldn't be denied those requested drinks of water and should be allowed to keep a water bottle at her desk.

Oxygen is, of course, critical to the brain. Higher levels of attention, mental functioning, and healing are linked to better quality air (less carbon dioxide, more oxygen). With only 36 percent of K-12 students in a daily physical education class, it is questionable whether they are getting enough oxygen-rich blood for highest performance. Movement and exercise are critical to learning—a concept that will be explored further in this chapter.

As professionals, we have been vastly underestimating the capacity of the learner. Our expectations have been too low for both the average and best of learners. It is important for educators to maintain high expectations in all children, regardless of diagnosed disabilities. Teaching material should be presented in many different learning styles so that the potential of every learner is accessed. Alternative forms of assessment should also be available to provide avenues of evaluation for those who learn differently. Classrooms should provide a climate in which every learner is respected and multi-status, multi-age, and multi-ability teamwork are utilized on a daily basis.

- **Gender**
  Healy, Epstein, and other scientists and developmental specialists have found that in the early years, brain growth rates may vary from as little as a few months to as much as five years. There are also definite differences in how the male and female brains develop. Whitleson says that boys show a much earlier specialization of the right brain than girls do. In a study of 200 right-handed children, the boys outperformed the girls on spatial tasks. But linguistically, the girls show earlier brain dominance than the boys. Because of right brain specialization, males have difficulty learning to read early in life.

Since reading is both spatial and linguistic, it makes sense that males learn to read later than females.

The brain not only grows differently in males and females, it also decays differently. We now know that the right brain of females has longer plasticity than that of males. This means it stays open to growth and change for more years in girls than in boys. Wree (1989) reports that the degeneration of nerve cells in the male brain precedes that of females by 20 years. Although the rate of the loss by females is greater than that of males, it is still not enough to overtake males in overall nerve cell degeneration. The researchers say that their estimates of cell loss are conservative.

There may be a reason why adolescent boys are more physically active than adolescent girls. The part of the brain that influences physical activity is much more developed in adolescent males. For females, the part of the brain used for interpersonal skills is more developed and plays an integral role in teenage girl culture.

The differences between males and females are so prevalent that same-sex teaching methods might need to be reconsidered. On the average, developmentally, girls read earlier than boys. If we actually accounted for differing brains, we'd suddenly find that 15-25% of all boys who are now considered "developmentally slow" would immediately be reclassified as "normal." Many male-female behaviors make much more sense when considered in the context of normal brain development.

Male and female brains not only act differently, but they are also structurally different. These verifiable physical differences may explain vastly different processing methodologies by male and female brains. Barrett (1992) says that the average male brain weighs 49 ounces and the average female brain weighs 44 ounces. Kimura (1989) says, "Taken altogether, the evidence suggests that men's and women's brains are organized along different lines from very early in life."

We may want to consider whether we have gone overboard in trying to make education "gender-bias free." Equal education does not mean that everything should be done the same; it means that it should provide equal opportunity. There are real, physical differences in male and female development that may need to be addressed in teaching styles.

Kimura (1992) says that males and females have very different ways of approaching and solving problems. She has been a pioneer for decades on the anatomical and functional differences between the sexes. Here is a summary of the research on differences in problem solving, broken down by gender. In general, females do better than males in the following areas:

✔ mathematical calculations
✔ precision, fine-motor coordination
✔ ideational fluency
✔ finding, matching, or locating missing objects
✔ use of landmarks to recall locations in context, maps

The problem-solving tasks that favor males are:

✔ target-directed motor skills (archery, football, baseball, cricket, darts, etc.)
✔ spatial; mentally rotating objects
✔ disembedding tests (locating objects, patterns from within another)
✔ mathematical reasoning, word problems
✔ use of spatial cues of distance, direction in route-finding

What this information suggests is that many problems may not be problems at all. They may simply be an expression of the "natural" way in which one sex or another really operates.

More males than females seem to exhibit ADD/ADHD behaviors, but the reason for this occurrence has not been identified. The average male brain follows the pattern of hemisphere specialization, while the female brain may diffuse more emotional processing across the two hemispheres (Moir, & Jessel, 1991). This organizational difference may help explain why males tend to restrict their language processing to the left hemisphere and most emotional processing to the right hemisphere. This neurologically explains why males tend to have more difficulty than females in talking about their feelings, and instead, express them through physical actions.

• **Environmental**
Many students who are thought of as being unmotivated or inattentive could become motivated or more attentive if they are provided with the right conditions. Current research is finding that environment does have an impact on

learning. Some researchers (Della Valle, Hodges, Shea, Kroon, 1986) have found that the classroom environment (seating choices, comfort levels, lighting) and learning styles (global, sequential, concrete, abstract, etc.) are significant factors in determining the success of students.

Ford (1992) researched optimal motivating environments and found that four factors were critical to what he calls "context beliefs." According to Ford, all of the following must be present to create an optimal environment:

1. The environment must be consistent with an individual's personal goals. This means that the learning environment must be a place in which the learner can reach his or her own personal goals.

2. The environment must be congruent with the learner's bio-social and cognitive styles. This means that if abstract learning is taking place in a crowded, competitive room with fluorescent lighting, it will be a problem for a concrete learner who needs space and works cooperatively.

3. The environment must offer the learner the resources needed. In addition to materials, advice, tools, transportation, and supplies, other key resources are time and affordability.

4. The environment must provide a supportive and positive emotional climate. Naturally, trust, warmth, safety, and peer acceptance are critical.

In another study, Desmond and Greenough (1991) conducted research using rats to investigate environmental impact. Their research drew three important conclusions:

1. Rats in enriched environments actually grew heavier brains with more dendritic connections that communicated better, increased synapses, greater thickness in sensory areas, increases in enzymes, and more glial cells (the ones that assist in growth and signal transmission).

2. The enriched environments needed to be varied and changed often to maintain the differences in rat intelligence. This meant larger cages, other rats, more toys, and frequent challenges.

3. Rats of any age could increase their intelligence if they were provided with challenging and frequent new learning experiences.

In working with children, Cain Ramey at the University of Alabama found that the results were similar to those found with rats. Ramey's intervention program worked with children of parents with lower IQs, who were divided into two groups. The children who were exposed to the enriched environment had significantly higher IQs than the control group. They were, in fact, 20 points higher. And the stronger results lasted; when the children were retested after 10 years, the effects of the early intervention had endured.

What this suggests is that we may be able to enhance brain growth and learning by altering the types of experiences offered. Speculation is that the most important influences for brain growth are interactive learning with novelty, unlimited choice, challenge, and learner-derived meaning from frequent new experiences.

Researchers Lozanov (1991), Nadel (1990), and Rosenfield (1988) have verified that the brain learns from both the traditional, focused kind of attention and from surrounding peripherals. They discovered that colors, decoration, sounds, smells and other stimuli are processed by the brain at a more subtle, nonconscious level. Yet they do influence the learner.

For example, different colors affect mood and learning. Calming colors are light blue and light green. Red is an engaging and emotive color best used in restaurants. For optimal learning, choose yellow, beige, or off-white. Those colors seem to stimulate positive feelings. Darker colors lower stress and increase feelings of peacefulness. Brighter colors, such as red, orange, and yellow, spark energy and creativity, but they can also increase aggressive and nervous behavior. The most neutral color is a textured, light gray. Teachers may be vastly underutilizing the potential of color in learning. Handouts should be on colored paper, overhead transparencies shouldn't be presented on stark white, and color should be used when designing mind maps for associative learning.

Rosenfield quoted a study done by Lozanov that used visual suggestion by color-coding key items. Five hundred subjects showed much greater recall than subjects who did not get the color-coded material. Peripherals in the form of positive posters; learner projects; and symbols of expression, change, growth, or beauty can be powerful. A classroom should be a happy, pleasant place to be. Furniture should be arranged in a way so that learners can see each other, which usually provides the most interesting visual enhancement of all.

In the *Brain-Mind Bulletin* (April, 1998), an article about Dr. Wayne London's experiments caught worldwide attention. London found that students who were in classrooms with full-spectrum lighting missed only 65% as many school days as those in other classrooms. London was not surprised. He said, "Ordinary fluorescent light has been shown to raise the cortisol level in the blood, a change likely to suppress the immune system."

What about bright versus dim lights? Many students relax, focus and actually perform better in low-light situations, says Krimsky, Dunn & Dunn, et al. Brighter lights, especially fluorescent, seemed to create restless, fidgety learners. Low-level lights seemed to have a calming effect, especially at younger ages. Many learners may be underperforming simply because the lighting is difficult on their eyes. More natural, brighter lighting is more conducive to learning.

Some learners perform better in a noisy, busy environment, while others need total silence. In one study (Carbo, Dunn & Dunn, 1986), 20% of learners preferred a noisy environment to a quiet one. On the other hand, some students need so much silence that only earplugs can filter out enough noise for their tastes. The use of music can also be quite powerful. Playing music while students are working and learning can be productive. A few students may complain that the music bothers them, but research suggests that the other 80-95% of the students will prefer to keep it on.

McCarthy (1991) says that even the amount of neatness and clutter in the learning environment varies by student. Teachers could be accidentally driving their learners crazy by stressing uniformity in the environment. It might be necessary to have separate environments or rotate the type used to accommodate different learning styles. Many learners could be underperforming because the environment doesn't suit their own, best learning style.

Room temperature is another consideration. A room that's cool for the teacher, could be hot for the learner. When students complain about room temperature, teachers are often perplexed. Some researchers (Della Valle, Hodges, Shea, Kroon, 1986) have found that the environment (seating choices, comfort levels, lighting) and learning styles (global, sequential, concrete, abstract, etc.) are a significant factor in determining the success of students. We may be creating learning environments that are too rigid. They may lack options for learners to sit where it's cooler or warmer, which might help their learning. Teachers might need to be more responsive to the classroom temperature as well as offering students choices for seating. It's better to be too cool than too warm, but the best is neither of these.

Seating options can also be a factor in learning. Dunn and Dunn (1987) say that at least 20 percent of learners are significantly affected, positively or negatively, based just on the type of seating options. To be at their best, students might need a choice. Some students need the floor, a couch, beanbag furniture, or even the option to stand.

Physical location in the classroom can also impact a student's success in the classroom. Wlodlowski (1985) says that circles, U shapes, and V shapes are best. When given a choice, good spellers tend to sit on the right side of the classroom. This may be related to handedness (hemispheric dominance), or left-brain-right field of vision, or the fact that visual creativity is dominant on the upper left side of the eye pattern range.

Sense of smell can also impact learning. There's a strong link between the olfactory glands and the autonomic nervous system. Olfaction (the neuroscience of smell) drives human basics, such as anxiety, fear, hunger, depression, and sexuality. Smell is an entire sense that has been underutilized in learning. Attention to the influence of aromas could be a very powerful strategy to reach some types of learners.

All this information supports the notion that teachers should consider the neurological stimulation present in a classroom setting, as it can enhance or hinder a student's ability to learn productively.

Learning Correlates in ADD/ADHD
Conditions for Powerful Learning
In general, we can say that people learn well under the following conditions:

What They Learn:
- ✔ is personally meaningful
- ✔ is challenging and they accept the challenge
- ✔ is appropriate for their developmental level

How They Learn:
- ✔ can learn in their own way, have choices, and feel in control
- ✔ use what they already know as they construct new knowledge
- ✔ have opportunities for social interaction
- ✔ get helpful feedback
- ✔ acquire and use strategies

Where They Learn:
- ✔ a positive emotional climate
- ✔ environment supports the intended learning

The Role of Attention in ADD/ADHD

Getting students' attention and keeping it has been the brass ring in the world of teaching. Many among us admire Hollywood teachers from movies like *Stand and Deliver, Dead Poets Society,* and *Dangerous Minds.* They rivet students' and our own attention, and we respect colleagues who can imitate their methods in real life. Attention has always been a central concern of educators. The brain's ability to focus and maintain its attention on objects and events is critical to learning and memory, and is a basic element in classroom motivation and management. ADD/ADHD significantly interferes with attention.

We tend to think about attention solely as a behavioral response to stimuli. If the stimuli present is emotionally of interest, then our attention should be maintained. It is important to re-orient to the biological factors that contribute to attention. Paying attention is not only a behavioral choice, it is also a neurological event. Can you recall attending a movie, play, or party when you really wanted to pay attention but were just too tired to maintain focus? The ability to sustain attention is partly chemical. If the neurological system is fatigued, attention will be impaired, regardless of the best intentions.

Until recently, cognitive scientists had only a limited understanding of the brain's attention mechanisms and processes, so educators had to rely on their own practical knowledge. This situation is rapidly changing as scientists unravel the mysteries of how and what to attend to, what to monitor, and what to ignore. Educators and parents must understand the basic mechanisms and processes that regulate attention for valid and effective application in the classroom and home.

Research has suggested that attention centers are located throughout the brain. The primary factors that determine attention are sensory input and chemicals produced in the brain in response to stimuli received. Contrasts in stimuli (e.g., movement, sound, smell) tend to trigger a stronger chemical response, hence heightened attention. The major influences for learning and attention are summarized in the following diagram.

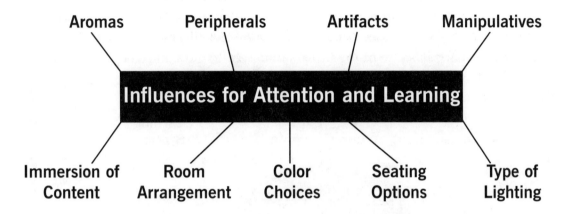

The pathway to attention consists of alarm, orientation, identification, and decision. This sequential, laser beam process is akin to, "Whoops, something's happening," then, "Where?" followed by, "What is it?" and finally, "What should I do?"

The process can be enhanced or hindered by the strength and pertinence of the stimulus presented. When specialized brain activity related to attention is activated, the person becomes alert and attentive. A greater flow of information in specific target areas of the brain's pathways is directly responsible for chemically turning on the brain to get and keep attention.

How does your brain know what specifically to pay attention to in the moment? The secret is that our visual system (which sends more than 80 percent of information to the brain in non-impaired learners) is not a one-way street. Information flows both ways, back and forth from our eyes, to the thalamus, to the visual cortex. This feedback is the mechanism that "shapes" our attention so that we can focus on one particular thing, like a teacher lecturing or reading a book (Kosslyn, 1992). Amazingly, the number of inputs that our "attention headquarters" gets as feedback *from* the cortex is nearly six times as high as the original input from the retina. That volume of feedback triggers certain selective neurons along the visual pathways to fire less often because their membranes are hyperpolarized to prevent normal processing. The appropriate way for attention areas to function means not just stimulating new neurons, but also suppressing unimportant information. Somehow, the brain corrects incoming images to help you stay attentive. What we see and attend to is a two-way balancing act of construction and feedback-maintenance of stimuli. The brain's susceptibility to paying attention is very much influenced by priming. We are more likely to see something if we are told to look for it or prompted to its location. The following chart summarizes some of the factors that help to gain and keep attention.

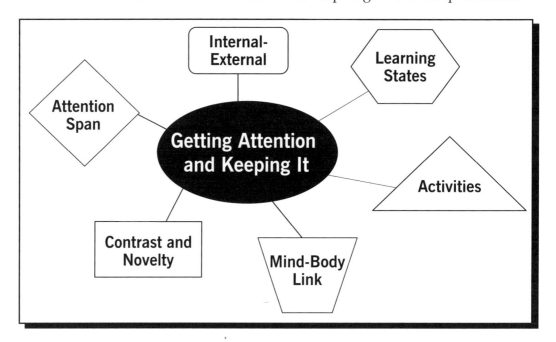

One factor that can positively influence attention is **choice**. Think about your day. Many people construct a list of things that need to be accomplished in a certain time frame. There may be tasks on the list that the person enjoys doing, and some other tasks that are not as pleasant. On some days, I like to tackle the unpleasant task first to get it out of the way and off the list so I can enjoy subsequent activities without the bad one hanging over my head. On other days, I might do everything on the list plus other tasks before I am ready to face the unpleasant one. The freedom to choose when I tackle certain tasks makes me more productive.

When a teacher has a daily list of things for a student with ADD/ADHD to accomplish, it might be beneficial to allow some choice in order of tasks. This allows the student to choose what they are ready to attend to and when to do it. When a required task is presented with no choice, the student may spend twice as much time and attention fighting the task than it would take to complete it if she were to approach it when in a prepared frame of mind.

A second factor that influences attention is **relevance**. Students are often asked to complete tasks simply because the teacher tells them to. Think about your own life. If your supervisor or spouse asks you to do a task that doesn't make sense and has no personal relevance for you, it is likely that you will make it a low priority or "forget" to do it altogether! The same can be true for the student with ADD/ADHD. If the functional reason for engaging in a task isn't clear, the child may give it minimal attention.

A third factor that influences attention is the **degree of personal involvement**. If a task engages the student in an active role, attention will be maintained longer. If the student is allowed a very passive role in learning, the attention factor will significantly decrease.

Another mistake that teachers make is to constantly require focused attention. We all tend to daydream and detour to personal tangents. Those short attention breaks actually work to improve saliency within learning. Constant attention can be counterproductive in a classroom setting. First, much of what we learn cannot be processed consciously; it happens too fast. We need time to process it. Second, in order to create new meaning, we need internal time. Meaning is always generated from within, not externally. Third, after each new learning experience, we need time for the learning to "imprint." It is important that we put our personal mark on it so that the new information is relevant to us personally.

An effective attention system must be able to do the following:
- ✔ quickly identify and focus on the most important items in the environment
- ✔ sustain attention while monitoring related information and ignoring other stimuli
- ✔ access memories that aren't currently active but could be relevant to the current focus
- ✔ shift attention quickly when important new information arrives

Two guiding principles for classroom management and instruction emerge from the current knowledge of attention. First, educators must adapt their instruction to the built-in biases of their students' innate attention mechanisms, and second, they should use imaginative teaching and management strategies to enhance the development of students' adaptable attention processes. Even though the scientific understanding of the attention system is fairly recent, successful teachers have grasped these principles of attention at a practical level. For example, many teachers learned to flip the light switch on/off to get students' attention. Teachers also instinctively knew that repetitive sedentary seat work needed to be followed by enjoyable activities that required more mental and physical energy. Another example is to schedule individualized subject skill areas in the morning and less precise, more social activities in the afternoon. Students' chemical levels for sustained precise attention are likely to be lower and students might be less alert in the afternoon.

The main challenge for educators is to help students learn how to consciously manage the adaptable aspects of their attention systems. It is important to teach students with ADD/ADHD to ignore certain comments and/or stimuli, while paying close attention to others. Cooperative learning activities help students stretch their attention by listening to contributions from a variety of individuals. Debates, discussion, role-play, simulations, storytelling, and games are all activities that require students to compare the real world with a created world and organize their thought processes.

The chart on the next page summarizes the average retention rate for learning in conjunction with types of educational activities.

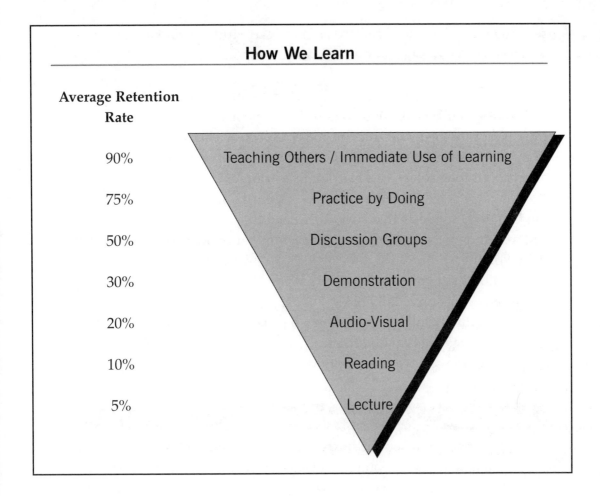

How We Learn

Average Retention Rate

90%	Teaching Others / Immediate Use of Learning
75%	Practice by Doing
50%	Discussion Groups
30%	Demonstration
20%	Audio-Visual
10%	Reading
5%	Lecture

Motivation and Learning

"…the behaviorists made a flawed assumption: that learning is primarily dependent on a reward. In fact, rats—as well as humans—will consistently seek new experiences and behaviors with no perceivable reward or impetus."

—Eric Jensen in *Teaching with the Brain in Mind*

How many of you persevered to achieve your chosen career in education because of the incredible financial rewards that it offers?! Well, then why did you choose this career? If you said things like, "I believe I make a difference; I enjoy children; I want summers off to do other things; I enjoy the challenges," then you just substantiated an internal intrinsic motivation for your learning. The external rewards of money, power, etc. were not the motivators you cited; however, in the educational system, teachers tend to rely on external artificial rewards to motivate students and are frustrated when students don't respond positively.

You have emotional, personal reasons for learning. That internal motivation influences your beliefs about yourself and what you stand for. The same must be approached with students today, especially children with ADD/ADHD. They need reasons, goals, and an internal motivation that allows them to feel good about themselves in a learning environment.

Jensen (1994) suggests that educators need to generate alternatives to external rewards and instead, promote intrinsic motivation in the classroom through the following:
- ✔ Eliminate threats.
- ✔ Set goals on a daily basis.
- ✔ Positively influence student's beliefs about himself and learning.
- ✔ Manage student emotions.
- ✔ Provide self-feedback options.

Eliminate Threats

Discover problems when they exist within a classroom. Avoid constantly making demands on students. Add time for transitions so students can accomplish closure on one subject before moving to the next. Don't introduce a topic or subject with negative consequences for non-effective learning; the student is threatened with failure before even beginning. Be careful of humiliating, finger-pointing, or using sarcasm to correct students. What will be remembered is the negative emotion, not the information. An embarrassed student isn't in a productive chemical state for learning!

Set Goals on a Daily Basis

Students who had a bad day yesterday don't need to be reminded of it at the beginning of the next day; instead, they need to feel that they can make a fresh start. Goals for the day should be set together with the child and teacher and they should be realistic and attainable. If a student with ADD/ADHD was in time-out ten times the day before, then the goal today should be nine or eight, not zero. Teachers should provide choices whenever possible to enhance motivation and neurological readiness to engage in a task. Provide reasons and a clear purpose for tasks rather than "because I said to do it." Make tasks meaningful and engage student emotions by telling why the task is important and relevant.

Positively Influence Student's Beliefs about Themselves and Learning

Alternate teaching strategies and presentation style to accommodate different learning styles and strengths/weaknesses. Use art, drama, music, physical education, and other adjunct interest areas to supplement subject skill drill with applied activities that incorporate the principles in an enjoyable situation. Use games and competition to increase teamwork and joint learning opportunities while enhancing individual motivation.

Manage Student Emotions

Create a positive environment in the classroom. Acknowledgement of successes should be frequent and maximized, with minimal class recognition of failures. Use rituals and routines to help a student learn a procedure through repetition to achieve success. Pair students with peers to encourage them to check on comprehension, compliance, etc. without feeling the spotlight on them by constantly bothering the teacher. Talk through negative reactions, outbursts, and teach alternative ways to vent and manage emotion. Award certificates for minimal positives to celebrate on-task occurrences. Students need to feel they can and are sometimes successful and productive in a classroom.

Provide Self-Feedback Options

Computer programs are structured to provide self-feedback without negative stigma attached. Projects are another way to channel learning without an obvious desired outcome that can be scrutinized by others for failure. Peers and family members can also be used to build self-feedback through discussion of learning and self-satisfaction with the outcome. Natural results should be emphasized as often as possible.

Movement and Learning

"Today's brain, mind, and body research establishes significant links between movement and learning. Educators ought to be purposeful about integrating movement activities into everyday learning."

—Eric Jensen in *Teaching with the Brain in Mind*

We know that the brain requires stimulation to develop. The brain can grow new connections in response to environmental stimulation within 48 hours. The process of making connections is what learning is all about! Increased neural stimulation results in increased neural connections. The brain can modify itself based on the type and amount of usage.

The *vestibular* (inner ear) and *cerebellar* (motor activity) systems are the first sensory systems to mature in humans. Consequently, movement and learning are intricately connected and cannot realistically be separated in young children. Sensory motor integration is fundamental to school readiness. We are finding that children of this generation have experienced more exposure to passive sedentary activities, such as video games, television, and videos, resulting in reduced neurological stimulation and development.

Research has repeatedly demonstrated the multiple benefits of exercise on learning. Among the leading beneficial aspects of exercise are the following:

- ✔ reduces stress
- ✔ fuels the brain with oxygen
- ✔ leads to increased connections among neurons
- ✔ triggers the release of chemicals that enhance cognition by improving the ability of neurons to communicate with each other
- ✔ increased alertness, attention, and relaxation

All of these aspects are critical to learning. The brain must be in a positive neurological state to effectively learn. Movement is one of the best ways to chemically boost the brain to an alert focused state.

Educators are beginning to understand the importance of movement on learning. The concept of learning centers in a classroom has been in effect for a long time, but the reason they worked so well is being substantiated now. Children learn by moving from place to place. The transition to a new location fires up the brain to become more receptive to the next learning task. Teachers are also inserting body energizers and stretch breaks between subjects to fuel the brain with more oxygen and pump the chemicals for better neurological communication. Allowing children to get up and move as they learn facilitates stronger memory traces for retention. A few examples for incorporating movement into learning are provided below.

✔ Have children rhythmically practice their spelling words with body movement. Have them clap out the letters, then stomp out the letters, then tap their thigh in rhythm to the letters. The body movement provides a stronger memory trace for those silent letters and vowel combinations than pure memorization.

✔ Math concepts are difficult to grasp for many children. Use body movement to clarify. For example, have children draw numbers from a basket and then line up in order from smallest to largest to teach number values, greater, less, etc. Have them measure objects in the room to get a practical sense of what an inch, foot, or yard really look like.

✔ Incorporate activities based on popular game shows (*Wheel of Fortune, Jeapordy!*, etc.) into teams for academic learning content.

✔ Use creative drama and role-play to have students re-enact their concept or understanding of major historical events. To teach the nuances of the court system, assign them all to a role and enact a trial.

It is critical that educators make a paradigm shift from behavior to neurology in addressing students with ADD/ADHD in a classroom. The challenges presented are not always under the conscious voluntary control of a student. Using natural neurological/chemical aspects to facilitate learning will help the student function more productively and feel better about herself in a learning environment.

Questions and Answers

How can I keep my student's attention?

Current research suggests that constant attention is not only impossible, but undesirable. The brain needs time for focusing and processing. Your students must first pay attention to the information being learned or discovered. Then they need time to make connections in their brains to form neural networks that lead to long-term memory.

Emotional stimulus and novelty are the two biggest attention-getters. It helps to keep these in mind when planning lessons. Another factor is biological. Our biochemistry runs in 90-minute cycles that fluctuate throughout the day. More attention neurotransmitters are available to us in the morning than in the afternoon (Sylwester, 1995). Perhaps that is why most primary teachers teach more difficult content in the morning and allow for more social interaction in the afternoon. This information should be a wake-up call for middle and secondary schools.

Another consideration is the brain's ability to pay attention. Research has found that the brain can direct its attention and block out another stimulus. In other words, if we direct our students to pay attention, they have more ability to do so. When we tell a student to "watch this carefully," a structure in the brain helps block out other stimuli and aids the occipital area in its focus.

What is an appropriate block of time to expect students to be able to learn?

Developmentally, the primary school brain learns best in shorter units of learning time—30-40 minutes in K-2 and 40-60 minutes in grades 3-5. The middle and high school learners are ready for, and need, class lengths in 90-150 minute blocks. This allows presenters and learners to better develop individual ideas. More importantly, it allows for the presenter-to-learner relationship that research has proven so valuable in productive learning situations.

What would one observe in schools/classrooms that practice brain-based theory?

Schools/classrooms would utilize more learning styles in the instructional process. Allowance would be given for differences in male and female brain development, differences for individual same-sex brain development. Teaching and assessing would utilize the theory of multiple intelligences. Stress threat and inappropriate discipline programs would be reduced or eliminated. Diversity is valued.

Chapter 6

Medical Intervention for ADD/ADHD

Case Example

José was very hyperactive. He woke up early in the morning and stayed active and up until late at night. He wandered off frequently, drawn by a squirrel or a dog that ran through the yard. He knew he wasn't supposed to leave the yard without telling me, but he just didn't seem to be able to control the immediate impulse to run after the animal that captured his attention. At school, the teacher complained constantly that José couldn't focus on anything for longer than a few minutes. His feet were continually tapping or swinging against the legs of his desk. His pencil was tapping out rhythms that disturbed other students. He drops his books, loses his papers, never can find his lunch ticket, and doesn't do assignments. We are at the emergency room monthly for stitches or X-rays for some injury. Yet José is a sweet little boy who is so soft-hearted and genuinely feels remorse for his actions, but he seems to forget almost immediately and the talks have no effect on "the next time." I don't want to use medication, but I am at my wit's end, and the teachers say he is in time-out or the principal's office more often than instruction. Help!

Following the diagnosis of ADD/ADHD, appropriate treatment options need to be pursued. Treatment of ADD/ADHD, like diagnosis, is not a simple, one-step process. Planning treatment will need to target identified deficits, and more than one intervention is often necessary.

For most children and adults with ADD/ADHD, medication is an integral part of treatment. Medication is not used to control behavior; medication is used to improve the symptoms of ADD/ADHD. The National Institute of Mental Health (NIMH) reports that methylphenidate (Ritalin) is the most frequently prescribed psychostimulant. Clinical trials have demonstrated its efficacy in controlling the symptoms of ADD/ADHD, with continuing beneficial effects as long as the medication is taken.

Nine out of ten professionals, including parents, believe that ADD/ADHD can have serious effects on children's academic performance and relationships if left untreated, yet the same percentage had apprehension about the use of medication to treat it (*Advance for SLP/A*, October, 2000). The same article reported that 92% of adults with ADD/ADHD who were first treated for the disorder at age 18 or above wished that they had been treated at a younger age. The adults with ADD/ADHD agreed that if the disorder is left untreated, it has serious effects on "work performance, career development, self-esteem, social skills, and relationships with family and co-workers." More than 90% of teachers, parents, physicians, and adults with ADD/ADHD agreed that medication was a successful treatment for controlling symptoms of ADD/ADHD.

Parent and teacher testimonials regarding the positive changes in response to medication are numerous.
- "Ritalin helped Henry focus and complete tasks for the first time."
- "Dexedrine helped Mark sit quietly, focus his attention, and participate in class so he could learn. He also became less impulsive and aggressive. Along with these changes in his behavior, Mark began to make and keep friends."
- "Everyone in the neighborhood has noticed the change in Sarah!"
- "Bobby used to wet the bed: now it doesn't occur at all."
- "How can two little pills change life so dramatically? Rachel is like a new person, both at home and school. She can sit still, she can write neatly, she doesn't tap her feet incessantly, and she actually told me what happened at school today in a coherent manner. She is being invited to birthday parties and over to friends' houses after school. I never thought I'd see the day!"

Unfortunately, when people see such immediate improvement, they often think medication is all that's needed; but medicines don't cure the disorder, they only temporarily control the symptoms. Although the drugs help individuals pay better attention and complete their work, they can't increase knowledge or improve academic skills. The drugs alone can't help people feel better about themselves or cope with problems. These require other kinds of treatment and support.

There is some debate as to whether Ritalin and other stimulant drugs are prescribed unnecessarily for too many children. Remember that many things, including anxiety, depression, allergies, seizures, or problems with the home or school environment can make children seem overactive, impulsive, or inattentive. Critics argue that many children who do not have a true attention disorder are medicated as a way to control their disruptive behaviors.

For lasting improvement, numerous clinicians recommend that medications be used in conjunction with treatments that address other aspects of the disorder. There are no quick cures. Many experts believe that the most significant, long-lasting gains appear when medication is combined with behavioral therapy, emotional counseling, and practical support. Some studies suggest that the combination of medicine and therapy may be more effective than drugs alone. Medication is never the only solution to treat ADD/ADHD; however, if no medication is considered, the optimal solution might not be in place.

Medication of children with ADD/ADHD remains controversial. Medication is not a cure and should not be used as the only treatment strategy for ADD/ADHD. While doctors, psychiatrists, and other healthcare professionals should be consulted for advice, ultimately a parent must make the final decision about whether or not to medicate a child.

Effective use of medication requires time, adjustment of dosage, and sometimes different medications or combinations. Reported short-term benefits of medication include a decrease in impulsive behavior, hyperactivity, aggressive behavior, and inappropriate social interaction, with an increase in concentration, academic productivity, and effort directed toward a goal. However, the long-term benefits of medication on social adjustment, thinking skills, and academic achievement are limited. These more applied areas of life require the implementation of other types of intervention to realize a positive effect.

If medication is chosen as an option, observe a child carefully for detrimental side effects. Some children lose weight, lose their appetite, or have problems falling asleep. Less common side effects include slowed growth, tic disorders, and problems with thinking or with social interaction. These effects can usually be eliminated by reducing the dosage or changing to a different medication.

The need for medication, type, and dosage can change as a child grows older. Many adolescents outgrow the need for medication, but it can be critical during the years between ages six to twelve in order to avoid significant problems in academic learning and social relationships with peers and family members.

Why Medication is Effective with ADD/ADHD

Scientists are laying a foundation for better understanding brain-related disorders of attention. Research continues to explore the neurological basis to ADD/ADHD. The results and impressions are allowing professionals to fine-tune intervention efforts within the medical realm. As research sorts out how a person mentally shifts attention from one subject or stimulus to another, deficits in attention can be better addressed. A study supported by the National Institutes of Health reported that individuals with ADD/ADHD have an impairment in the brain structures that allow for control of attention (*Advance for SLP/A*, August, 1999).

The primary neurological structure involved in research on ADD/ADHD for many years was the Reticular Formation, or Reticular Activating System, which is in the brainstem. The reticular formation serves as a sensory switching system for the brain. Stimuli collected by the peripheral nervous system (eyes, ears, nose, mouth, skin, limbs, etc.) are sorted and directed to appropriate cortical areas for response at the level of the reticular formation. This structure makes a preliminary decision as to whether a stimulus is important for focused cortical attention or can be responded to with a more automatic reflex. The reticular formation is also the alerting, or arousal, mechanism for the upper cortex, telling the brain to wake up and pay attention to incoming stimuli. The reticular formation is thought to be hyperactive to incoming stimuli, resulting in poor sorting and directing to the brain. Too much stimuli is sent to the cortex, resulting in confusion and a conscious decision on the individual's part as to what stimulus they should pay attention to. Switches in attention occur in cortical areas and can be monitored by specially modified magnetic resonance imaging (MRI) scanners.

At present, scientists believe that the major problem in the attention centers of the brain in a person who has the diagnosis of ADD/ADHD is a difference in the dopamine system. Current research shows that there may be as many as 13 different genes that vary from the so-called normal genes, resulting in what are called "attention deficits." These genes, which are called alleles because they are alternatives to the most common variety of gene, are mainly involved with the dopamine system. The gene differences create a decreased amount of dopamine to support the system and allow it to work in a consistent and predictable manner. The behavioral result is poor focused attention for a sustained or organized effort by the individual.

Consequently, the treatment for ADD/ADHD rests on the drugs that are known to affect the dopamine system: the stimulants, the antidepressants, and precursors that may boost the effectiveness of dopamine. While most neuroscientists are hesitant to explain any multi-faceted disorder with a simple equation, it does appear that attention problems may be best interpreted as a dopamine deficiency. Thus the job of medication is to correct this deficit and its associated problems, such as anxiety, depression, emotionality and mood changes, overactive startle response, and problems associated with aggression and addiction. The medication increases dopamine in certain parts of the brain where it is being inadequately produced or utilized.

The U.S. Food and Drug Administration (FDA) recently approved a medication for ADHD that is not a stimulant. The medication, Strattera®, or atomoxetine, works on the neurotransmitter norepinephrine, whereas the stimulants primarily work on dopamine. Both of these neurotransmitters are believed to play a role in ADHD. More studies will need to be done to contrast Strattera with the medications already available, but the evidence to date indicates that over 70 percent of children with ADHD who have been given Strattera demonstrate significant improvement in their symptoms.

Many physicians feel that medication should be the first line of treatment because the brain is not working correctly. Behavior modification should be the second line. To some, the philosophy of trying behavior modification before medication is like punishing a child for having ADD/ADHD. Giving medication allows the brain to respond better to behavior and learning strategies.

It is important for parents and professionals to understand and acknowledge that there is a neurological basis for ADD/ADHD. When medication is used, it is an attempt to "normalize" or improve the biochemical levels of the individual with ADD/ADHD to make him more productive. While behavioral strategies can have positive effects, it is important that medication not be ruled out as a treatment option. It is consistent with the etiology of the disorder and may be the most effective in turning around a child's life.

Medication Considerations and Issues

While many professionals agree that the use of medications can substantially benefit children with ADD/ADHD, there are no hard and fast rules as to when medication should be administered. The decisions to medicate should be made with consideration of several factors:

1. *Age of Child*
    Generally, medications to treat ADD/ADHD are less effective with children below the age of five than they are for older children. Also younger children seem to exhibit greater side effects.

2. *Use of Non-Medical Interventions*
    The utilization of non-medical interventions such as educational accommodations, parent training, and brain-based teaching strategies may be useful to pursue prior to the use of medication. Such interventions may eliminate or decrease the need for medication.

3. *Risk of Side Effects*
    No medication prescribed is without potential side effects. Prior history of motor tics or the presence of severe anxiety, for example, may rule out the use of medication. Before considering medication, one should always ask whether the benefits outweigh the risks for a particular child.

4. *Opinion of the Teacher*
    Teachers should be surveyed for their opinions as to a student's need for medication. Classroom behavior can be significantly different than characteristics observed at home, due to increased structure and academic demands.

5. *Concerns of the Parents*
    Parents should be educated about ADD/ADHD and the various treatments available before making any decision regarding the use of medications. Such a decision is important and should be made in conjunction with other professionals.

The specific dose of medicine must be determined for each individual. There are ranges based on a medication dose per unit of body weight that are usually employed; however, there are no consistent relationships between height, age, and clinical response to a medication. A medication trial is often used to determine the most beneficial dosage. The trial usually begins with a low, weight-based dose that is gradually increased until clinical benefits are achieved. It is common for the dosage to be raised several times during the trial. The patient is monitored both on and off the medication. For children, observations are collected from parents and teachers, even coaches and tutors. Parent and teacher rating scales are often used. In the case of an adult, the patient and significant family members share their impressions with the treatment team.

Stimulant drugs, such as Ritalin, Cylert, and Dexedrine, when used with medical supervision, are usually considered safe. They seldom make children "high" or jittery, nor do they sedate a child. Rather, the stimulants help children control their hyperactivity, inattention, and other behaviors. However, the issue of co-morbidity with other disorders, such as Oppositional Defiant Disorder, can lead to a tendency to later misuse of medication and needs to be carefully monitored.

As useful as drugs are, Ritalin and the other stimulants have sparked a great deal of controversy. Most doctors feel the potential side effects should be carefully weighed against the benefits before prescribing the drugs. While on these medications, some children lose weight, have less appetite, and temporarily grow more slowly. Others may have problems falling asleep. Some doctors believe that stimulants may also make the symptoms of Tourette's syndrome worse, although recent research suggests this may not be true. Other doctors say that if the child's height, weight, and overall development are carefully monitored, the benefits of medication far outweigh the potential side effects. Side effects that occur can often be handled by reducing the dosage.

Different doctors use the medications in slightly different ways. Cylert is available in one form, which naturally lasts five to ten hours. Because of its potential for serious side effects affecting the liver, Cylert should not ordinarily be considered as a first-line drug therapy for ADD/ADHD. Ritalin and Dexedrine come in short-term tablets that last about three hours, as well as longer-term preparations that last through the school day in a time-release format. The short-term dose is often more practical for children who need medication only during the school day or for special situations, like attending church or studying for an important exam. The sustained-release dosage frees the child from the inconvenience or embarrassment of going to the office or school nurse every day for a pill. However, parents should be cautioned that medication should be administered consistently, not only when a structured situation is scheduled. The doctor can help decide which preparation to use and whether a child needs to take the medicine during school hours only or in the evenings and on weekends. It is important to realize some children require medication benefits to cope with structured settings, while others need medication year-round to manage social behavior and everyday activities.

Nine out of ten children show discernable improvement when taking one of the three stimulant drugs, so if one doesn't help, others should be tried. Usually a medication should be taken for at least one week to see if positive changes result. If necessary, the doctor can make adjustments in the dosage before switching to a different medication.

Other types of medication may be used if stimulants don't work or if the ADD/ADHD occurs concomitant with another disorder. Antidepressants and other medications may be used to help control accompanying depression or anxiety. In some cases, antihistamines can be tried. Clonidine, a drug normally used to treat hypertension, may be helpful in people with both ADD/ADHD and Tourette's syndrome. Although stimulants tend to be more effective, Clonidine can be tried when stimulants aren't effective or can't be used. Clonidine can be administered either by pill or by skin patch and has different side effects than stimulants.

The prescribing doctor must work closely with each patient to find the most appropriate medication. Sometimes a child's ADD/ADHD symptoms seem to worsen, leading to questions as to why. Parents should be assured that a drug that helps rarely stops working; however, they might need to work with the doctor to make sure that the child is getting the right dosage. Professionals with questions should always make sure that a child is actually taking the prescribed daily dosage at home and/or at school—it's easy to forget. Parents also need to know that new or exaggerated behaviors may appear when a child is under stress. The challenges that all children face, like changing schools or entering puberty, may be even more stressful for a child with ADD/ADHD.

Some doctors recommend that a child be taken off a medication now and then to see if she still needs it. They recommend temporarily stopping the drug during school breaks and summer vacations when focused attention and calm behavior are usually not as crucial. These "drug holidays" work well if the child can still participate at camp or other activities without medication.

Children on medications should have regular check-ups. Parents should also talk regularly with the child's teachers and doctor about how the child is doing. This is especially important when a medication is first started, re-started, or when the dosage is changed. It's natural for parents to be concerned about whether taking a medicine is in their child's best interests. Parents need to be clear about the benefits and potential risks of using drugs. The child's pediatrician or psychiatrist can provide advice and answer questions.

Medication Options

The two primary routes for medication management of ADD/ADHD symptoms are the use of stimulants and antidepressants. While other options are available, these are the most common treatments initiated. The following section provides information on these two treatment options, followed by a summary chart of other medication options.

Stimulants

"Psychostimulant" compounds are the most widely used medications for the management of ADD/ADHD-related symptoms. It is believed that psycho-stimulant medications change the levels of transmitter chemicals available to various neurotransmitter systems in the brain. These neurotransmitters are the means by which the different nerve cells communicate among themselves. Between 70-80% of children with ADD/ADHD respond positively to these medications. Attention span, impulsivity, and on-task behavior improve, especially in structured environments. Some children also demonstrate improvements in frustration tolerance, compliance, and even handwriting. Relationships with parents, peers, and teachers may also improve.

Psychostimulant medication can also be effective in adults with ADD/ADHD. The reaction to these medications can be similar to that experienced by children with ADD/ADHD—a decrease in impulsivity and an increase in attention. Many adults with ADD/ADHD treated with psychostimulant medication report that they are able to bring more control and organization to their lives. Other medications, such as antidepressants, can be helpful when depression, phobic, panic, anxiety, and/or obsessive-compulsive disorders are present.

Common psychostimulant medications used in the treatment of ADD/ADHD include methylphenidate (Ritalin), single-entity amphetamine products (Adderall), and dextroamphetamine (Dexedrine—including one brand with several related compounds). Ritalin and Adderall-type medications are short-acting, while Dexedrine and others are longer-acting medications. The effects of methylphenidate, for example, usually last for about four hours. The effects of a longer-acting psychostimulant medication like dextroamphetamine can last for up to eight hours, though there can be wide individual variation that cannot be predicted and will only become evident once the medication is tried.

Hundreds of studies on thousands of children have been conducted regarding the effects of psychostimulant medications, making them among the most studied medications in pharmacological history. Unfortunately, there are no good long-term studies on the use of psychostimulant medications. Each family must weigh the pros and cons of choosing medication as part of the treatment plan for ADD/ADHD. Most immediate side effects related to these medications are mild and typically short-term. A few of the common effects are summarized below:

✔ The most common side effects are reduction in appetite and difficulty sleeping.

✔ Some children experience "stimulant rebound"—a negative mood or an increase in activity when medication is losing its effect. This tends to occur in younger children and is usually seen as a short-acting medication wears off (frequently just as the child arrives home from school). If the child continues to exhibit signs of rebound after about two weeks, the doctor should be consulted. These side effects are usually managed by changing the dose and the scheduling for short-acting medications, or by changing to a prolonged-release formulation.

✔ There may be an initial, slight effect on height and weight gain, but studies suggest that ultimate height and weight are rarely affected.

✔ Some studies suggest that children with ADD/ADHD reach puberty later than their peers. However, for any child who seems to be lagging behind his or her peers, height and weight should be closely monitored.

✔ A relatively uncommon side effect of psychostimulant medications may be the unmasking of latent tics—the medical term for involuntary motor movements, such as eye blinking, shrugging, and clearing of the throat. Psychostimulant medications can facilitate the emergence of a tic disorder in susceptible individuals. Often, but not always, the tic will disappear when the medication is stopped. For many mid-teenagers, vocal tics (throat clearing, sniffing, or coughing beyond what is normal) or motor tics (blinking, facial grimacing, shrugging, head-turning) will occur as a time-limited phenomenon concurrent with ADD/ADHD. The medications may bring them to notice earlier, or make them more prominent than they would be without medication. Eventually these tics will go away in the latter part of the teenage years, even while the individual is still on medication.

Myths About Stimulant Medication

Myth: **Stimulants can lead to drug addiction later in life.**

Fact: Stimulants help many children focus and be more successful at school, home, and play. Avoiding negative experiences early in life may actually help prevent addictions and other emotional problems later.

Myth: **Responding well to a stimulant drug proves a person has ADD/ADHD.**

Fact: Stimulants allow many people to focus and pay better attention, whether or not they have ADD/ADHD. The improvement is just more noticeable in people with ADD/ADHD.

Myth: **Medication should be stopped when the child reaches adolescence.**

Fact: Not so! About 80% of those who needed medication as children still need it as teenagers. Fifty percent need medication as adults.

Anti-Depressants

Medications initially developed as antidepressants are used less frequently for ADD/ADHD than stimulant medications, but they have been shown to be effective with some children. Those antidepressants that have active effects on the neurotransmitters—norepinephrine and dopamine (the tricyclic classes, and novel medications like Buproprion) can have an effect on ADD/ADHD. They are used when contra-indications to psychostimulant medications exist, when psychostimulant medications have been ineffective, or when unacceptable side effects have resulted.

Antidepressants that affect the neurotransmitter serotonin (the serotonin selective reuptake inhibitors, or SSRIs) have no effect on ADD/ADHD, but they may be effective against co-existing conditions. Clonodine, originally an antihypertensive medication, is also being prescribed for some children with ADD/ADHD, though its effect seems to be primarily on intrusive and hyper-active behavior, rather than on selective attention.

A summary chart of medications commonly prescribed to improve behaviors associated with disposition for learning is provided on the next page. Medications to address ADD/ADHD are often encompassed under this category. Beneficial effects (+) and possible side effects (-) are included, as well as typical age for prescription initiation.

Medications Commonly Prescribed
to Improve Behavior, Mood, and Learning

Category	Medications (Approved Age)	Therapeutic (+) Effects And Side (-) Effects
Psychostimulants	Ritalin® (6+) Dexedrine® (3+) Desoxyn® (3+) Adderall® (3+) Dextrostat® (3+) Cylert® (6+) (Note: Due to its potential for serious side effects affecting the liver, Cylert should not ordinarily be considered as first line drug therapy for ADD/ADHD.)	(+) May reduce impulsivity, increase attentional strength, diminish motor activity, enhance certain memory functions. (-) May cause tics, loss of appetite, growth delays, sleep problems, personality change; Cylert may disrupt liver function.
Tricyclic Antidepressants	Anafranil® (10+ for OCD) Effexor® (18+) Tofranil® (6+ for bed-wetting) Sinequan® (12+)	(+) May reduce anxiety, depressive symptoms, aggression, overactivity, obsessive-compulsive signs. (-) May cause sedation, changes in heart rhythm, gastro-intestinal disturbance.
Aminoketones	Wellbutrin® (18+)	(+) May reduce hyperactivity, anxiety and aggressive tendencies. (-) May cause insomnia, headaches, gastro-intestinal distress, seizures.
Mood Stabilizing Medications	Lithium (12+) Eskalith® (12+) Depakote® (2+ for seizures) Tegretol® (Any age for seizures)	(+) May be effective in bipolar illness (manic-depression); may also help in depression when other drugs fail. (-) May cause gastro-intestinal upset, tremor, weight gain, urinary symptoms, poor motor coordination.
Anti-psychotic Agents	Haldol® (3+) Mellaril® (2+) Seroquel® (18+) Zyprexa® (18+) Orap® (12+ for Tourette's—data for age 2+ indicate similar safety profile)	(+) May help attention in low doses, reduce tics in Tourette syndrome, lessen aggressive symptoms. (-) May be overly sedative, interfere with cognition and learning, cause movement disorder (tardive dyskinesia).
Alpha-Adrenergic	Clonidine (Catapres®) Guanfacine (Tenex®) (Note: The use of these drugs in children is off label. Safety in children has not been established.)	(+) May increase frustration tolerance, reduce impulsivity, improve task oriented behaviors in children with motoric over-activity, lessen tics in Tourette syndrome, improve sleep. (-) May overly sedate, cause fall in blood pressure, induce depression or other mood disorder.

Physician's Desk Reference, 52nd ed., Medical Economics Data Production Company, Montavie, N.J.,1998.

"Practice Parameters for the Assessment and Treatment of Children, Adolescents and Adults with Attention Deficit/Hyperactivity Disorder," Journal of American Academy of Child and Adolescent Psychiatry, Vol. 36(10), October 1997.

Taylor, M., "Evaluation and Management of Attention-Deficit Hyperactivity Disorder," American Family Physician, Vol. 55 Num. 3, 1997, pp. 887-894.

Levine, Melvin D., *Developmental Variation and Learning Disorders*, Educator Publishing Service, Inc., Cambridge and Toronto, 1993.

A summary chart of medications commonly prescribed to specifically address ADD/ADHD is summarized below. All of the medications listed are in the psychostimulant category. The "Approved Age" column indicates that the medication has been tested and found to be safe and effective in children of the specified age.

Medications Commonly Prescribed for ADD/ADHD

Trade Name	Generic Name	Approved Age
Adderall	amphetamine	3 and older
Concerta	methylphenidate (long acting)	6 and older
Cylert*	pemoline	6 and older
Dexedrine	dextroamphetamine	3 and older
Dextrostat	dextroamphetamine	3 and older
Focalin	dexmethylphenidate	6 and older
Metadate ER	methylphenidate (extended release)	6 and older
Metadate CD	methylphenidate (extended release)	6 and older
Ritalin	methylphenidate	6 and older
Ritalin SR	methylphenidate (extended release)	6 and older
Ritalin LA	methylphenidate (long acting)	6 and older

*Because of its potential for serious side effects affecting the liver, Cylert should not ordinarily be considered as first-line drug therapy for ADHD.

Monitoring Medication in the Classroom

Between 60 and 90 percent of students with ADD/ADHD are treated with some form of medication. Due to legal issues, a teacher should not specifically recommend medication. The teacher should share behavioral and/or academic observations, and work with the team to discuss strategies that could address issues of concern. One option available to parents is to consider taking the child to a doctor for an examination.

As discussed in Chapter 4, the diagnosis of ADD/ADHD is more likely to be introduced within the school setting. The physician's role is to assist the parents and child with medical options to manage disruptive characteristics. Medical personnel are the only individuals who can actually prescribe medication.

If medication is prescribed by a doctor, the school should be informed about the type of medication prescribed, when the medication is to be taken, and what side effects might develop. A proper dose of medication should not make a child sleepy or lifeless, but should enable a child to focus on his work without being easily distracted.

While medication can reduce children's hyperactive behavior temporarily, it does not solve the academic problems experienced by children with ADD/ADHD, and most studies show that medication has few long-term benefits to academic achievement and social adjustment. Instead, medication is a tool that facilitates the use of other methods for helping students with ADD/ADHD. For example, a child will complete more work when the child's academic schedule is coordinated with the medication so that most of her schoolwork can be finished while the medication is calming the child's behavior. A child should not take medication without an adult present, and the school's policy may require the school nurse to administer the medicine. The school or parents should inform all of the child's teachers about the medication so they can be alert for side effects and medical problems.

Once medication therapy has begun, it is extremely important to take steps to monitor the effects of the medication on the child. Schools play an ever-increasing role in providing concrete feedback regarding the effects of medication on children. The **Assessing Medication Effectiveness** checklist on page 116 can be used to evaluate both unwanted side effects as well as main effects that the child may experience as a result of medication treatment.

Medication and Self-Esteem

When a child's schoolwork and behavior improve soon after starting medication, the child, parents, and teachers tend to applaud the drug for causing the sudden change. But these changes are actually the child's own strengths and natural abilities coming out from behind a cloud. Giving credit to the medication can make the child feel incompetent. The medication only makes these changes possible. The child must supply the effort and ability. To help children feel good about themselves, parents and teachers need to praise the student, not the drug.

It's also important to help children and teenagers feel comfortable about a medication they must take every day. They may feel that because they take medicine they are different from their classmates or that there is something seriously wrong with them. C.H.A.D.D. (i.e., Children and Adults with Attention Deficit Disorders), a leading organization for people with attention disorders, suggests several ways that parents and teachers can help children view the medication in a positive way:

- Compare the pills to eyeglasses, braces, and allergy medications used by other children in their class.
- Explain that the medicine is simply a tool to help them focus and pay attention.
- Point out that they're lucky their problem can be helped.
- Encourage them to identify ways the medicine makes it easier to do things that are important to them, like make friends, succeed at school, and play.

Ultimately, the success of an individual with ADD/ADHD depends on a collaborative effort between the child and a committed team of caregivers. Medication provides an opportunity for the multi-dimensional treatment program to be effective and can maximize the effects of other interventions. Taken alone, however, medication is often not enough to help.

Medication can help control some of the behavior problems that lead to family turmoil. But more often, there are other aspects of the problem that medication can't touch. Even though ADD/ADHD primarily affects a person's behavior, having the disorder has broad emotional repercussions. For some children, being scolded is the only attention they ever get. They have few experiences that build their sense of worth and competence. If they're hyperactive, they're often told they're bad and punished for being disruptive. If they are unable to complete tasks due to being disorganized and unfocused, others may call them lazy. If they impulsively grab toys, interrupt, or shove classmates, they lose friends. And if they have a related conduct disorder, they may get in trouble at school or with the law.

Facing the daily frustrations that can come with having ADD/ADHD can make children fear that they are strange, abnormal, or stupid. Often, the cycle of frustration, blame, and anger has gone on so long that it will take some time to undo. Both parents and children may need special help to develop techniques for managing existing patterns of behavior. In such cases, mental health professionals can counsel the child and family, helping them develop new skills, attitudes, and ways of relating to each other. In individual counseling, a therapist helps children or adults with ADD/ADHD learn to feel better about themselves. They learn to recognize that having a disability does not reflect who they are as a person. The therapist can also help people with ADD/ADHD identify and build on their strengths, cope with daily problems, and control their attention and aggression. In group counseling, people learn that they are not alone in their frustration and that others want to help. Sometimes only the individual with ADD/ADHD needs counseling support. But in many cases, because the problem affects the family as well as the individual with ADD/ADHD, the entire family may need help coping. The therapist assists the family in finding better ways to handle the disruptive behaviors and promote change. If the child is young, most of the therapist's work is with the parents, teaching them techniques for managing and improving their child's behavior.

It is important that a child with ADD/ADHD not experience only negative reinforcement. Inappropriate behaviors are likely to escalate when the only time a child is successful in gaining attention is for negative behavior. It is important to find strengths and positive aspects of a child's personality and aptitudes and capitalize on those. Individuals must experience positive feelings about themselves before other treatment effects can be maximized.

Other Medical-Based Intervention Options

Several intervention approaches are available, and different therapists tend to prefer one approach or another. Knowing something about the various types of medical-based treatments can make it easier for families to choose an intervention plan and professionals that are right for their needs.

- *Psychotherapy* works to help people with ADD/ADHD like and accept themselves despite their disorder. In psychotherapy, patients talk with the therapist about feelings and upsetting events and thoughts to explore self-defeating patterns of behavior and learn alternative ways to handle their emotions. As they talk, the therapist tries to help them understand how they can change. However, people dealing with ADD/ADHD usually want to gain control of their symptomatic behaviors more directly. If so, more direct kinds of intervention are needed.

- *Cognitive-behavioral therapy* helps people work on immediate issues. Rather than helping people understand their feelings and actions, it supports them directly in changing their behavior. The support might be practical assistance, like helping Joshua learn to think through tasks and organize his work. The support offered might be to encourage new behaviors by giving praise or rewards each time the person acts in the desired way. A cognitive-behavioral therapist might use these techniques to help a belligerent child learn to control fighting, or an impulsive teenager to think before she speaks.

- *Social skills training* is another treatment that can help children learn new behaviors. In social skills training, the therapist discusses and models appropriate behaviors like waiting for a turn, sharing toys, asking for help, or responding to teasing, and then gives children a chance to practice the new behavior. For example, a child might learn to "read" other people's facial expressions and tone of voice in order to respond more appropriately. Social skills training can help children learn to join in group activities, make appropriate comments, and ask for help. It can also help aggressive students learn to understand how their behavior affects others and develop new ways to respond when angry or pushed.

- *Support groups* connect people who have common concerns. Many adults with ADD/ADHD and parents of children with ADD/ADHD find it useful to join a local or national support group. Members of support groups share frustrations and successes, referrals to qualified specialists, and information about what works, as well as their hopes for themselves and their children. There is strength in numbers, and sharing experiences with others who have similar problems helps people know that they aren't alone.

• *Parenting skills training,* offered by therapists or in special classes, provides parents with tools and techniques for managing their child's behavior. One such technique is the use of "time-out" when the child becomes too unruly or out of control. During time-outs, the child is removed from the agitating situation and sits alone quietly for a short time to calm down. Parents may also be taught to give the child "quality time" each day, in which they share a pleasurable or relaxed activity. During this time together, the parent looks for opportunities to notice and point out what the child does well, and praise his strengths and abilities.

An effective way to modify a child's behavior is through a system of rewards and penalties. The parents (or teacher) identify a few desirable behaviors that they want to encourage in the child, such as asking for a toy instead of grabbing it, or completing a simple task. The child is told exactly what is expected in order to earn the reward. The child receives the reward when he performs the desired behavior and a mild penalty when he doesn't. A reward can be small, perhaps a token that can be exchanged for special privileges, but it should be something the child wants and is eager to earn. The penalty might be removal of a token or a brief "time-out." The goal, over time, is to help children learn to control their own behavior and to choose the more desired behavior. The technique works well with all children, although children with ADD/ADHD may need more frequent rewards.

In addition, parents may learn to structure situations in ways that will allow their child to succeed. This may include allowing only one or two playmates at a time, so that their child doesn't become overstimulated. Or if a child has trouble completing tasks, they may learn to help the child divide a large task into small steps, then praise the child as each step is completed.

Parents may also learn to use stress management methods, such as meditation, relaxation techniques, and exercise to increase their own tolerance for frustration so that they can respond more calmly to their child's behavior.

Controversial Treatments for ADD/ADHD

Parents are eager to help their children with ADD/ADHD and, understandably, want to explore every possible option. Recent innovations in treatment provide an increased variety of options for parents. Many sound reasonable, some come with glowing anecdotal reports, while others are extremely questionable. While some are developed and advocated by reputable doctors or specialists, they cannot be scientifically proven to make a difference. Despite that fact, it is worthwhile for parents and professionals to be informed so they can make a decision regarding the treatment options available for individuals with ADD/ADHD.

- *Dietary Intervention*
  Over the years, proponents of the Feingold Diet have made many dramatic claims. They state that the diet, which promotes the elimination of most additives from food, will improve most (if not all) children's learning and attention problems. In the past 15 years, dozens of well-controlled studies published in peer-reviewed journals have consistently failed to find support for the Feingold Diet, while a few studies have reported some limited success with this approach. At best, empirical research suggests that there may be a small group of children who are responsive to additive-free diets. At this time, it has not been shown that specialized or restrictive dietary intervention offers significant help to children with learning and attention problems.

- *Megavitamins and Mineral Supplements*
  The use of very high doses of vitamins and minerals to treat ADD/ADHD is based on the theory that some people have a genetic abnormality that results in increased requirements for vitamins and minerals. Although vitamins are virtually synonymous with health, there is a lack of supporting scientific evidence for this treatment. There are no well-controlled studies supporting the claims; for the studies in which proper controls were applied, none reported positive results. Both the American Psychiatric Association and the American Academy of Pediatrics have concluded that the use of megavitamins to treat behavioral and learning problems is not justified.

- *Anti-Motion Sickness Medication*
  Advocates of this theory believe that there is a relationship between ADD/ADHD and problems with coordination and balance that can all be attributed to problems in the inner-ear system, which plays a major role in balance and coordination. This approach is not consistent with what is

currently known about ADD/ADHD, and it is not supported by research findings. Anatomically and physiologically, there is no reason to believe that the inner-ear system is involved in attention and impulse control other than in marginal ways regarding vestibular stimulation.

• *Candida Yeast*
Advocates of this model believe that toxins produced by yeast overgrowth weaken the immune system and make the body susceptible to ADD/ADHD and other psychiatric disorders. There is no evidence from controlled studies to support this theory, and it is not consistent with what is currently known about the etiology of ADD/ADHD.

• *EEG Biofeedback*
Proponents of this approach believe that children with ADD/ADHD can be trained to increase the type of brain-wave activity associated with sustained attention and to decrease the type of activity associated with daydreaming and distraction. Several studies have produced impressive results, but these studies are seriously flawed by the use of small numbers of children with ambiguous diagnoses and the lack of appropriate control groups. This is an expensive, unproven approach, and parents are advised to proceed with caution.

• *Applied Kinesiology*
Advocates of this approach, also known as the Neural Organization Technique, believe that learning disabilities are caused by the misalignment of two specific bones in the skull which creates unequal pressure on different areas of the brain, leading to brain malfunction. This theory is not consistent with either current knowledge of the etiology of learning disabilities nor knowledge of human anatomy, as even standard medical textbooks state that cranial bones do not move. No research has been done to support the effectiveness of this form of treatment.

• *Optometric Vision Training*
Advocates of this approach believe that visual problems (e.g., faulty eye movements, sensitivity of the eyes to certain light frequencies, focus problems), cause reading disorders. Scientific studies of this approach are currently few in number and flawed in design. In 1972, a joint statement highly critical of this optometric approach was issued by the American Academy of

Pediatrics, the American Academy of Ophthalmology and Otolaryngology, and the American Association of Ophthalmology. In the absence of supporting evidence for its effectiveness, this approach should not be employed in the treatment of learning disabilities. Parents are advised to proceed with caution.

- *Glyconutrients*
  The use of glyconutrients as a treatment for ADD/ADHD is based on the hypothesis that the disorder is due to an auto-immune system dysfunction. Glyconutrients are a food supplement that is added to provide eight glycoproteins to a child's diet. The premise is that a child lacks essential proteins, which adversely impact neural function, the ability to think, attend, and cognitive development. The supplement provides essential carbohydrates to prevent poor immune system function, thereby avoiding or remediating the multitude of disorders that can result.

In summary, anecdotal stories of success shouldn't replace or substitute for scientific evidence when making treatment decisions. Until sound, scientific testing shows a treatment to be effective, families risk spending time, money, and hope on fads and false promises. In the area of medication and other chemical intervention, side effects can be serious and should never be tried on a child with ADD/ADHD without physician consultation.

Questions & Answers

What are the suggested treatment strategies for ADD/ADHD?

There is no fixed approach as to what will work and what will be the most effective with every child. Treatment may be a combination of medical interventions, parent and teacher training, accommodations in the regular classroom, special education and/or related services, counseling, and behavioral management strategies. Remember, not all individuals with ADD/ADHD are alike, and treatment approaches must be decided on an individual basis.

Why is it sometimes necessary to treat ADD/ADHD with prescribed drugs?

Researchers believe that ADD/ADHD is a neurobiological problem caused by neuro-transmitters that are not working properly. A 1990 study by Dr. Alan Zametkin established a biochemical link to ADD/ADHD. Because ADD/ADHD has a biochemical basis, medication is frequently prescribed to enhance functioning of neurotransmitters, the chemical messengers of the brain. The three neurotransmitters most commonly associated with ADD/ADHD are norepinephrine, dopamine, and serotonin. The medications most commonly prescribed for ADD/ADHD all affect the production or absorption of neurotransmitters.

As a parent, what can I do to ensure the effectiveness of any medication prescribed for my child diagnosed with ADD/ADHD?

To be effective, medications for ADD/ADHD must be used properly. Parents need to discuss with the physician any questions they have about medication. Take a notebook with you to the doctor's visit. Have your questions written down and write down answers. Parents need to be sure to administer the medication appropriately. Observe and record your child's responses to medication. Never stop, increase, or decrease the dosage of medication without consulting the doctor. Talk to your child about the medication. Teach the child that taking the medication is a responsibility. Explain to the child what the medication is and is not for. Ask the child if he has any questions. Share information with the child's caregivers and teachers. Explain that the medication is long-term and your child's help is needed in monitoring side effects. Provide clear instructions for giving the child medication if a dose is to be given while the child is away from home. Follow up and make sure the medication was given.

Are medications for ADD/ADHD being overprescribed?

If ADD/ADHD is incorrectly diagnosed, then medication may be overprescribed. Chapter 2 discussed the other disorders often associated with ADD/ADHD, and Chapter 4 discussed the need for a multi-faceted approach to the diagnosis of ADD/ADHD. There have been studies in a variety of states that focused on the prescribing practices of medication for ADD/ADHD. A summary of findings from a 1987 study in Maryland, a 1990 study in Virginia, and another study have indicated no evidence of widespread abuse. There has, however, been a dramatic increase in the distribution of medication for ADD/ADHD over the last decade. Appropriate diagnosis, planning, treatment, and monitoring are essential to reduce potential misuse of any medication.

As a teacher, what are some things I need to know about medication and ADD/ADHD?

Teachers have increased responsibility for students who are taking medication for management of ADD/ADHD. You will often be asked to provide the physician with a detailed description of the student's school adjustment and behavior. You may also help the physician monitor the effects and side effects of the medication on the student's behavior in school, reporting any changes to facilitate adjustments to the medication dosage. School personnel may also be required to administer medication. Make sure you have a clear record of dosage, administration, and responsibility guidelines spelled out in the child's school file.

Is Ritalin a dangerous drug?

The use of the stimulant medication Ritalin for ADD/ADHD has been known since 1937. There is extensive research over more than fifty years showing that it is an effective medication for ADD/ADHD and that it is a safe drug. As with any drug, there are some potential side effects. These were discussed earlier in this chapter. Ritalin, when used for correctly diagnosed ADD/ADHD and when monitored properly, is a safe and effective medication.

Assessing Medication Effectiveness

Child's Name:		Age:	Date:

Current Medication(s)   **Medication Initiation Date**

1. _____   _____

2. _____   _____

3. _____   _____

Medication Effectiveness	Teachers should complete this form to determine changes in behavior within the school setting. Circle the number that best describes the child.					

Positive Behaviors	Strongly Disagree	Disagree	No Change	Agree	Strongly Agree	Comments (Optional)
1. Improved academic performance	1	2	3	4	5	
2. Receives passing grades	1	2	3	4	5	
3. Completes homework	1	2	3	4	5	
4. Completes assignments	1	2	3	4	5	
5. Pays attention in class	1	2	3	4	5	
6. Participates in class	1	2	3	4	5	
7. Obeys school rules	1	2	3	4	5	
8. Gets along with peers	1	2	3	4	5	
9. Stays awake in class	1	2	3	4	5	
10. Listens when others talk	1	2	3	4	5	
11. Obeys authority figures	1	2	3	4	5	

Negative Behaviors	Strongly Disagree	Disagree	No Change	Agree	Strongly Agree	Comments (Optional)
1. Is easily distracted	1	2	3	4	5	
2. Is forgetful	1	2	3	4	5	
3. Is irritable	1	2	3	4	5	
4. Is aggressive	1	2	3	4	5	
5. Is impulsive	1	2	3	4	5	
6. Talks back to adults and peers	1	2	3	4	5	
7. Is easily frustrated	1	2	3	4	5	
8. Is constantly moving	1	2	3	4	5	

Name of person completing form:	Position:

Chapter 7

Behavioral Intervention for ADD/ADHD

Case Example

Teacher's Side: I'm not a novice teacher, but I sure feel like I am with A.J. He is always one step ahead of me and in trouble before I can even set the rule. His behavior swings are driving me crazy! He goes from aggressive anger to genuine tears in seconds. He can't understand why he's always in time-out, yet he pushes all the buttons to end up there several times throughout the day. I feel like I should just reserve the chair for him. Nothing I do works to keep him controlled and compliant with classroom rules. Either he goes or I go!

Parent's Side: The school says they can't handle A. J. anymore. I've tried all kinds of discipline at home and I understand their frustration. I hate to admit it, but I've even tried spanking him; it doesn't seem to have any effect. The school says the only option left is a behavior-disorders placement. He's not a bad kid. He's just very active and doesn't think before he says or does something. I don't know how to get through to him, so I guess I can't blame the school. But I don't think putting him in a classroom surrounded by discipline problems is going to help; it will probably get worse because he will become friends with those kids.

Child's Side: My parents and teachers are always yelling at me. They find fault with everything I do. I can't turn around without them saying I have to go sit in time-out. When I'm there, I don't really know what I'm supposed to do, so I just get madder. I wish they'd just tell me what they want me to do so I could do it. Most of the time I'm just trying to have a little fun! What's wrong with that?!

Managing Behavior in ADD/ADHD

The ability to effectively manage behavior in children with ADD/ADHD is one of the greatest challenges for parents and teachers. The crux of the problem lies in how children with ADD/ADHD respond to environmental stimuli. Often they tend to over-respond, resulting in the appearance that they can't even handle normal situations in an appropriate way. What should be positive stimulation ends up triggering negative reactions. Consequently, parents and teachers throw up their hands in exasperation of "having tried everything."

- **SPC: Simple, Positive, Clear Approach**
  Believe it or not, "everything" hasn't been tried! Sometimes we simply need to be more creative and innovative in the way we approach behavior management with ADD/ADHD. The attitude in which parents or professionals approach behavior management makes a difference. If the child perceives that you have given up and feel it is hopeless before even starting, then it is! A simple, positive, clear approach often has the best results rather than the elaborate systems that are often established.

  The "Special" approach, abbreviated as SPC: Simple, Positive, Clear.

  ✔ **Simple**
  An effective behavior management system concentrates on a few behaviors at a time, with additional behavior patterns added when the first ones are mastered. A common mistake is in trying to address all the problematic behaviors at once, resulting in total confusion for the child. When children complain that they don't know what they did wrong, they really don't because there are so many "don'ts" included in the system. The behavior management system must focus on a few behavior targets at first and ignore the others until later.

  ✔ **Positive**
  Children with ADD/ADHD respond well to a behavior management system in which rewards are given for good behavior. Reward systems encourage students to work toward earning privileges or rewards by gaining points for desired behavior. Some systems also incorporate losing points for undesirable behavior with the positive. If you use this system with younger children, you may want to make charts or use tokens or stickers to show students the consequences and positive results of their behavior. The critical aspect is that the system not focus only on the negative.

  It's also important that the reinforcement be something the student is willing to work for (or to avoid). The teacher needs to give or remove tokens/points immediately, according to the behavior, so the child understands why he is being rewarded or punished. While older children may be willing to work toward a deferred reward, younger children will require immediate concrete reinforcement.

✔ **Clear**

You can help children with ADD/ADHD behave in a disciplined manner in the classroom by establishing a few rules that result in immediate consequences when they are broken. Give the child specific rules that are phrased positively in terms of what the child should do. When you praise and reward the student for good behavior and punish for inappropriate behavior, the child can see you apply the rules fairly and consistently.

Another proven strategy teachers use is to provide a specified time-out location where the student can go when she is not in control. This should not be seen as a punishment but as a place for the student to go for a few minutes to calm down. Older students can be taught to sense when they are getting out of control and go to the time-out area on their own.

Since children with ADD/ADHD have difficulty understanding different rules for different places, parents and teachers benefit from working together to develop a consistent set of rules and a similar management system. When teachers and parents communicate with each other about a child with ADD/ADHD, they increase the likelihood that she will be able to learn effectively.

• **Behavior Analysis**
Professionals have learned that observing a behavioral response can actually occur for a variety of reasons. It is important that a teacher not assume to know the cause of a behavior without taking the time to further analyze the situation. The teacher must carefully assess the function or reason a child is evidencing such a behavior. If the teacher addresses the behavioral symptom only, the behavior is likely to occur again. On the other hand, if the teacher evaluates the reason the behavior occured, intervention can address the cause more productively and the need for the inappropriate symptomatic response can be discontinued.
Behavior analysis is designed to help a parent or professional focus on

identifying biological, social, environmental, or other reasons underlying a behavior. This type of assessment allows an evaluator to go beyond the symptom and discover the "why" for a student's misbehavior.

Behavior analysis does not suggest that the child's misbehavior should be justified or accepted. Rather it is an attempt to determine if the student could learn a different behavior to replace the inappropriate one he is demonstrating. In fact, the replacement behavior would serve the same function or motivation for the student but in a more appropriate manner. Behavior analysis allows professionals to develop strategies to circumvent inappropriate student behaviors by identifying the reasons a particular behavior occurred and teaching an alternate, better behavioral response.

For this reason, behavior must always be evaluated in the contextual situation in which it occurred. Successful analysis of behavior requires assessment of cognitive, social, emotional, and environmental factors that contribute to the circumstances that trigger a behavioral response. It often requires discussion with other team members and sometimes the student to accurately determine the reasons underlying a behavior. The biggest stumbling block is a tendency for a professional to "read into" a behavior and assume she knows the reason without objectively exploring circumstances. However, if careful objective observation is completed, behavior can be addressed very successfully.

The concept of **SPC** is incorporated into behavioral analysis. The decision to be made regarding an observed behavior is whether it occurred for one of the following reasons:

S kill Deficit

P erformance Deficit

C ompliance Deficit

✔ **Skill Deficit** suggests that a child with ADD/ADHD is lacking knowledge of a certain required skill, resulting in an inappropriate behavioral response. Students who haven't developed certain skills or knowledge in specific areas often exhibit inappropriate behaviors that cover their embarrassment or help them avoid or escape the task for which they are unprepared. When trying to analyze whether a behavior could be caused by a skill deficit, evaluators should ask themselves if the child understands the situation and its behavioral expectations. What behavioral skills are required, and does the child possess those or has he learned what is expected?

✔ **Performance Deficit** occurs frequently in ADD/ADHD due to the nature of the disorder. This is when the child has the knowledge of what to do in a situation, but he has failed to read the environmental cues necessary to prompt the appropriate behavioral response. Impulsivity, hyperactivity, and other components of ADD/ADHD contribute greatly to behavior problems associated with performance deficits. Sometimes a child has the knowledge or skill but is uncertain about how to actually respond in a certain situation.

✔ **Compliance Deficit** is when a child has the skills, has processed environmental cues and controlled impulsive responses, and simply makes a poor choice. This is when a child consciously decides to test limits and misbehave.

If careful, objective behavioral analysis has been completed, then the behavior management plan should become obvious.

For *skill deficits*, the student needs to be taught appropriate behavioral responses to implement in certain situations. Specific, clear goals should be devised to **Teach** deficit social, academic, communication, or emotional knowledge. The outcome will be appropriate responses when the student with ADD/ADHD has the knowledge and skills to respond to situations with understanding, competence, and confidence.

Performance deficits require **Accommodation** strategies in the school or home settings to assist the student in making more appropriate choices. A performance deficit implies that the child with ADD/ADHD knows the skills necessary to demonstrate an appropriate behavioral response, but he does not consistently use that knowledge. Therefore, the behavior plan is to provide techniques, strategies, and supports designed to overcome the deficits associated with ADD/ADHD.

Compliance deficits are not unusual; all children test limits at times. It is important to give a child with a disability the same parameters to test those limits. However, for students with ADD/ADHD, principles of **Positive behavior management** should be implemented. This will allow the child to respond to motivation, rewards, and incentives to make more appropriate choices regarding conscious behavior decisions.

This behavioral approach can be summed up as **"TAP into SPC."**

Teach   **S**kill Deficit

Accommodation   **INTO**   **P**erformance Deficit

Positive Behavior Management   **C**ompliance Deficit

A chart to assist in evaluating behavioral responses using this system is included on the following pages. The possible observed behaviors are further classified into groups of academic, social interaction, communication/language, and emotional areas. This will help define the area of specific skills to teach, accommodate, or intervene with positive behavior management techniques. Remember, don't assume. Instead, objectively explore causes for behavior! The form on the following pages is a quick, efficient way to analyze behaviors that easily translates into a behavior management plan. A sample completed form and discussion are included, beginning on page 126.

TAP into SPC

Child's Name:			Date of Observation:
Person Completing Form:			Observation Setting:

Observation **Academic**	**Skill Deficit**	**Performance Deficit**	**Compliance Deficit**
Not listening			
Disorganized			
Not paying attention			
Not following directions			
Not completing assignments			
Not turning in assignments			
Forgetful; poor memory			
Careless			
Rushes through assignments			
Interaction	**Skill Deficit**	**Performance Deficit**	**Compliance Deficit**
Not following rules			
Creating distractions			
Not staying in seat			
Immaturity			
Not able to transition			
Not accepting consequences			
Poor peer interaction			
Poor adult interaction			
Impulsive			
Physically active			
Not accepting authority			
Poor tolerance of others			
Unable to share			
Takes items without permission			
Damages others' possessions			
Late / tardy			
Poor hygiene			
Noncompliant			
Difficulty waiting			
Poor turn taking			
	Teach	**Accommodate**	**Positive Behavior Management**

TAP into SPC, *continued*			
Observation			
Communication	**Skill Deficit**	**Performance Deficit**	**Compliance Deficit**
Inappropriate verbal outbursts			
Not seeking assistance			
Rude			
Poor conversation skills			
Lies /fabricates stories			
Asks irrelevant questions			
Observation			
Emotional	**Skill Deficit**	**Performance Deficit**	**Compliance Deficit**
Inappropriate physical outbursts			
Inappropriate anger			
Gets in fights			
Not tolerating teasing			
Not tolerating criticism			
Poor loser			
Minimal remorse			
Resistance to consequences			
Oversensitive/over-reactive			
Blaming others			
	Teach	**Accommodate**	**Positive Behavior Management**

- **Directions for Using "TAP into SPC"**
  The person observing the child should not necessarily be engaged in
  intensive teaching with the child or class. It is important for the observer
  to concentrate on behavioral characteristics and be able to make judgments regarding the underlying reason for their occurrence. Completion
  of the chart simply requires putting an "X" or check mark in the column
  that best explains the reason for an observed behavior. A section of the
  chart is reproduced below and examples provided.

TAP into SPC			
Child's Name: Chandler Jones		Date of Observation: 9-27-01	
Person Completing Form: Ann Pace, LD Teacher		Observation Setting: 3rd Grade Class	
Observation **Academic**	**Skill Deficit**	**Performance Deficit**	**Compliance Deficit**
Not listening	X		
Disorganized		X	
Not paying attention	X		
Not following directions		X	
Not completing assignments			
Not turning in assignments			
Forgetful; poor memory			
Careless			
Rushes through assignments			

The Learning Disabilities Resource teacher observed Chandler in the regular third grade classroom. The classroom teacher was involved in a verbal
lesson on math. Chandler was gazing out the window (behavior = not
paying attention/not listening). As the teacher continued the lesson,
Chandler did not seem to understand what was being presented and did
not have his book open to the right page to follow along (behavior = not
following directions). He had a pencil but no paper to write problems as
the teacher demonstrated on the board (behavior = disorganized).

This very brief observation already resulted in four behaviors listed in the
first section (academic) on the chart. As the teacher noted the behavior,
she needed to make a judgment as to whether Chandler was not paying
attention and not listening. Her conclusions are listed on the next page.

✔ He didn't understand.	*skill deficit*
✔ He couldn't focus due to ADD/ADHD.	*performance deficit*
✔ He didn't want to pay attention.	*compliance deficit*

His disorganization and lack of following directions as the teacher was instructing the class could have been due to the following:

✔ poor understanding/comprehension	*skill deficit*
✔ impulsivity/distractibility of ADD/ADHD	*performance deficit*
✔ conscious choice not to get out his pencil	*compliance deficit*

The teacher observing might want to mark the behaviors with a small check in the left margin, and then after observing a bit longer to get better impressions, make an X in the actual column that she thinks the behavior represents.

The behaviors are then approached according to deficit area. For example, the teacher now presumed that Chandler's lack of focused attention and listening was due to the fact that he found the content of the math lesson confusing and unclear (skill deficit). Perhaps Chandler has a learning disability that has impacted math. Time-out, telling him to pay attention, or refocusing him won't resolve the behavior. He needs to understand the lesson to pay attention better. Intervention needs to address teaching him the math concepts to understand class material.

Secondly, the teacher interpreted Chandler's disorganization and lack of following directions to write the problems due to his ADD/ADHD characteristics (performance deficit). Consequently, accommodations should be implemented, such as having a folder with all materials (paper, pencil eraser, book) for each subject in it to help keep Chandler organized.

The other behaviors were not observed, so no marks were made.

If careful, objective charting of behavioral responses is completed, then intervention should be more effective for both the child with ADD/ADHD and the professional involved in remediation. In this way, meaningless punishments or unrealistic demands are not placed on a child, setting him up for failure.

It will not always be possible to determine with certainty the actual reason or cause for a behavioral occurrence. The observer should simply do the best she can. It is possible that check marks are by behaviors as having been observed (left side of form), but an "X" into a specific column for judgment/interpretation isn't provided. That is okay and realistic for some behaviors, but it is important that a decision not be avoided for all of the behaviors observed. Otherwise, the direction of intervention will also be undetermined. Careful observation leads to effective intervention, which makes everyone happier!

Specific Behaviors and Suggestions for ADD/ADHD

It is impossible to list all possible behaviors or concerns associated with the disorder of ADD/ADHD. However, one of the best learning techniques is to talk through some specific examples to illustrate the idea of SPC—specific, positive, and clear. A summary chart of specific behavioral examples can be found on the following pages, followed by some suggestions for approaching that behavior.

Common Behaviors of Children with ADD/ADHD

Challenging Behaviors	Possible Interventions
• Seeks independence and freedom	• Encourage independence. • Trust until proven untrustworthy. • Be observant of activities & friends. • Set up win-win situations. • Offer an attractive alternative.
• Disobeys/conflicts with adults	• State rules clearly. • Involve in developing rules. • Write down rules/post them.
• Acts younger/immature	• Teach desired behavior. • Adjust expectations. • Impose consequence if necessary.
• Acts impulsive	• Anticipate problems. • Consider medication. • Discuss/model appropriate behavior.
• Difficulty paying attention/ Doesn't seem to listen	• Make eye contact/use touch. • Keep instructions brief & simple. • Avoid "preaching." • Give instruction in writing. • Have child repeat directions.
• Forgetful/Doesn't complete assigned tasks	• Make a written list. • Use Post-it® notes. • Help get started/show how to do. • Impose consequences.
• Disorganized/loses things/ messy room	• Put name on possessions. • Offer incentives. • Assist in being organized. • List steps for task completion. • Close door to messy room.
• Lacks awareness of time/ always late	• Use a wrist watch alarm. • Rent or buy a beeper. • Teach awareness of time.

Common Behaviors of Children with ADD/ADHD, *continued*

Challenging Behaviors	Possible Interventions
• Seek material possessions	• Allow to earn money. • Plan for holidays or birthdays. • Express gratitude.
• Self-centered	• Model helping others. • Encourage to do things for others. • Discuss other peoples' perspectives.
• Breaks things	• Maintain composure and calmness. • Discuss valuing others' property. • Put expensive possessions away.
• Daring/has accidents/ does harrowing stunts	• Encourage safe stimulating activities. • Monitor level of danger. • Provide supervision.
• Sleep disturbances/ can't fall asleep	• Establish reasonable bedtime. • Prompt to get ready for bed. • Establish bedtime routine. • Don't start projects after set time. • Encourage exercise during the day. • Consider medication/confer with Dr.
• Can't wake up	• Buy alarm clock. • Connect lights and TV to timer. • Try positive incentives. • Look for other causes.
• Difficult morning routine	• Allow enough time. • Use logical consequences; walk to school; leave on time/dress in car; give 10 minute warning; take away privileges. • Get things ready the night before. • Use checklist of steps for morning routine.

Common Behaviors of Children with ADD/ADHD, *continued*	
Challenging Behaviors	**Possible Interventions**
• Difficulty planning ahead	• Teach planning. • Teach time management.
• Difficult to discipline	• Use positive reinforcement. • Use logical consequences. • Be consistent. • Create new consequences/rewards. • Use behavioral charts. • Use rewards. • Avoid power struggles. • Redirect interests.
• Low frustration tolerance/ Irritable/emotional	• Listen/be supportive. • Teach problem-solving skills. • Teach anger control.
• Argues/talks back	• Ignore minor infractions. • Walk away from conflict. • Give space and time to cool off. • Impose a consequence.
• Doesn't accept responsibility for actions	• Implement behavior plan. • Impose natural consequences.
• Dishonest	• Teach and discuss honest behavior. • Develop plan to deal with problem. • Impose a consequence.
• Difficulty with family events	• Keep outings simple/reduce demands. • Discuss expected behaviors.
• Difficulty participating in sports	• Play large muscle sports. • Play an active position. • Consider individual exercise/sports.
• Restless/easily bored	• Participate in activities and sports. • Plan interesting activities. • Encourage hobbies & interests. • Structure free time.

As a child with ADD/ADHD matures, the typical adolescent characteristics can further complicate the behaviors previously mentioned. The following chart summarizes some of the unique behavioral challenges a teen with ADD/ADHD faces.

Behaviors Unique to Teens with ADD/ADHD	
ADD	
• Lethargy/apathy	• Encourage physical activity. • Consult physician. • Get physical exam. • Check for depression/meds if needed.
• Absent-minded/spacey	• Implement organizational strategies. • Anticipate problems/make adjustments. • Medication may help.
• Slow processing	• Make adaptations. • Implement school modifications. • Allow additional time.
ADD/ADHD	
• Attention seekers	• Give opportunities to be center stage. • Participate in activities allowing recognition. • Discuss inappropriate attention. • Ignore some behavior.
• Intrusive	• Set boundaries. • Identify parent's & sibling's space. • Impose consequences. • Teach to wait.
• Difficulty relating to others	• Invite friends on outings. • Provide tips on relating to friends. • Wait for teachable moment. • Encourage having friends of both genders.

Pragmatic / Social Behaviors

Certain social competencies are necessary for a child to experience academic and emotional success. As mentioned previously in this chapter, many children with ADD/ADHD demonstrate deficit behaviors due to a lack of knowledge. There are many excellent social skills programs now available to teach functional social skills in applied settings with children across the age spectrum.

It is important to realize how much depends on awareness of social expectations for students to succeed in school. A list summarizing possible skills to evaluate and teach students with ADD/ADHD is provided in the following section. For the **Teach** and **Accommodate** columns on the "Tap into SPC" behavioral analysis chart, any of these could be the actual goal to address for a child with ADD/ADHD.

Social Competencies for Children with ADD/ADHD

Skills for the Classroom

listening	asking for help
saying thank-you	bringing materials to class
following instructions	completing assignments
contributing to discussions	offering help to an adult
asking a question	ignoring distractions
making corrections	deciding on something to do
setting a goal	

Skills for Making Friends

introducing yourself	beginning a conversation
ending a conversation	joining in
playing a game	asking a favor
offering help to a classmate	

Skills for Dealing with Feelings

dealing with anger	dealing with another's anger
expressing affection	dealing with fear
rewarding yourself	

Skills for Dealing with Stress

dealing with boredom	deciding causes of problems
making a complaint	answering a complaint
dealing with losing	showing sportsmanship
dealing with being left out	dealing with embarrassment
reacting to failure	accepting no
saying no	relaxing
dealing with group pressure	making decisions
being honest	dealing with wanting something that isn't mine

Skills for the Alternatives to Aggression

using self-control	asking permission
responding to teasing	avoiding trouble
staying out of fights	problem solving
accepting consequences	dealing with accusation
negotiating	

Another way to address interpersonal relationships is to identify the area of skill deficit and in **simple, positive, clear** language, specify the objective or goal to address the deficit area. Some examples are provided in the following section.

Accepting Authority

- to comply with request of adult in position of authority
- to comply with request of peer in position of authority
- to know and follow classroom rules
- to follow classroom rules in the absence of the teacher
- to question rules that may be unjust

Coping with Conflict

- to respond to teasing or name calling by ignoring, changing the subject, or some other constructive means
- to respond to physical assault by leaving the situation, calling for help, or some other constructive means
- to walk away from a peer when angry to avoid hitting

- to refuse the request of another politely
- to express anger with nonaggressive words rather than physical action or aggressive words
- to handle constructive criticism or punishment perceived as undeserved

Gaining Attention

- to gain teacher's attention in class by raising hand
- to wait quietly for recognition before speaking out in class
- to use "please" and "thank you" when making requests of others
- to approach teacher and ask appropriately for help, explanation, instructions, etc.
- to gain attention from peers in appropriate ways
- to ask a peer for help

Greeting Others

- to look others in the eye when greeting them
- to state one's name when asked
- to smile when encountering a friend or acquaintance
- to greet adults and peers by name
- to respond to an introduction by shaking hands and saying "how-do-you-do?"
- to introduce oneself to another person
- to introduce two people to each other

Helping Others

- to help teacher when asked
- to help peer when asked
- to give simple directions to a peer
- to offer help to a teacher
- to offer help to a classmate
- to defend a peer in trouble
- to express sympathy to a peer about problems or difficulties

Making Conversation

- to pay attention in a conversation to the person speaking
- to talk to others in a tone of voice appropriate to the situation
- to wait for pauses in a conversation before speaking
- to make relevant remarks in a conversation with peers
- to make relevant remarks in a conversation with adults
- to ignore interruptions of others in a conversation
- to initiate conversation with peers in an informal situation
- to initiate conversation with adults in an informal situation

Organized Play

- to follow rules when playing a game
- to take turns when playing a game
- to display effort in a competitive game
- to accept defeat and congratulate the winner in a competitive game

Positive Attitude Toward Others

- to make positive statements about qualities and accomplishments of others
- to compliment another person
- to display tolerance for persons with characteristics different from one's own

Play Informally

- to ask another student to play on the playground
- to ask to be included in a playground activity in progress
- to share toys and equipment in a play situation
- to suggest an activity for the group on the playground

Care of Property

- to distinguish one's own property from the property of others
- to lend possessions to others when asked
- to use and return others' property without damaging it
- to ask permission to use another's property

Accepting Consequences

- to report to the teacher after spilling or breaking something
- to apologize when actions have injured or infringed on another
- to accept deserved consequences of wrongdoing

Ethical Behavior

- to distinguish truth from untruth or fantasy in one's own statements
- to answer truthfully when asked about a possible wrongdoing
- to identify consequences of behavior involving wrongdoing
- to avoid doing something wrong when encouraged by a peer

Expressing Feelings

- to describe one's own feelings or moods verbally
- to recognize and label moods of others

Positive Attitude Toward Self

- to say "thank you" when complimented or praised
- to be willing to have one's work displayed
- to make positive statements when asked about one's self
- to undertake a new task with a positive attitude

Responsible Behavior

- to be regular in school attendance
- to arrive at school on time
- to hang up one's clothes in a required place

Attitude for Approaching Behavior Management

In *Survival Kit for Teachers and Parents, 2nd Ed.* (Collins & Benjamin, 1993), a series
of 28 beliefs are listed in the beginning of the book. These statements articulate
the attitude in which teachers and parents must approach behavior management.
Extrapolating from those beliefs, we have compiled a list of ten thoughts to focus
professionals and parents as they generate behavior management ideas.

- Teachers and parents are intelligent beings who can generate positive and
  innovative suggestions toward behavior management.

- Concentrate on past successes rather than failures. Parents and teachers
  will discover a repertoire of successful strategies if they work collabora-
  tively.

- No one technique will work all the time with any student. Allow ineffective instances before abandoning a strategy.

- The best behavior management techniques are preventive, proactive
  strategies, rather than reactive ones.

- To help a child, the teacher or parent must recognize the behavior as an
  SOS or signal for help. The teacher and parents must believe the behavior
  is a distress call for help, not an opportunity for punishment.

- No behavior is by chance: there is a reason for behavior. Good management strategies should explore reasons for behavior occurrence and then
  explore alternative choices.

- The humane goal is to help students achieve enhanced self-esteem and
  personal dignity. A person who feels good about himself will exercise
  self-discipline. Participation and responsibility are prerequisites to self-
  discipline. Involve the child in development of the behavior management
  system to accomplish these goals.

- Utilization of extrinsic rewards to modify behavior does not prevent the
  student from developing intrinsic values. Teachers and parents whose
  values are clearly modeled are better able to help students work through
  conflicts and confusion.

- Consistent behavioral expectations are critical in maintaining an environment conducive to learning. Learning is not a singular experience: it is a
  composite of facts, skills, and attitudes.

- Whatever is done reinforces behavior in one way or another. A behavior
  management approach must be functional and pragmatic. Children do
  not learn well when embarrassed, ashamed, or stressed. Respect and positive reinforcement must be the overriding factors in any approach to learning appropriate behavior responses.

Applying Behavior Modification Strategies with ADD/ADHD

A child with ADD/ADHD typically has multiple behaviors of concern that are interwoven, creating a complex problem to address—where do you start? Professionals in the school setting usually have some training in the principles of behavior management. It is important to use the formula previously introduced (SPC) to break down the behavioral issues into manageable, specific parts. Consequently, most behavioral plans require coordination between parents and school personnel, but are first established in the school setting.

Parents can implement a simplified version of a behavior modification plan utilized in the school setting; however, it is important for the team in conjunction with the parents to determine the variables that work effectively. Some modified versions of behavioral plans for home implementation are included in the Home Intervention chapter (Chapter 9).

A behavioral approach to modifying problematic characteristics of ADD/ADHD requires a sequenced, coordinated plan. The steps recommended are outlined below and then explained in more detail in the following section. It is important that the steps be implemented as a team or in cooperation with all individuals who interact with the child.

- Observe, analyze, and measure behaviors.
- Identify target behaviors for modification.
- Identify positive reinforcements and incentives.
- Identify contingencies or consequences to be used in conjunction with positive incentives.
- Apply strategies to decrease inappropriate behaviors and increase appropriate behaviors.

✔ **Observe, analyze, and measure behaviors.**
Teachers and parents must learn how to concretely identify problem behaviors and avoid talking about behavioral concerns in generalities. For example, a teacher reports that the student with ADD/ADHD never pays attention in class. This description defies realistic modification. The teacher needs to define what behaviors are being summarized to her conclusion of not paying attention. Does the student stare out the window, fidget in her seat, play with her pencil, or gaze absently into space? The time frame and subject areas for not paying attention also need to be more definitely described. Is the child distracted by outside noises, is attention

better at the beginning of a lesson than at the end, at what point does fidgeting behavior become noticeable? Behavior modification can only be successful if behaviors are specifically defined.

It is also important to determine for whom the behavior is a problem. Does the behavior create danger for anyone? Does the behavior impede learning for other students? What is the impact of the behavior? Sometimes teachers and parents have unrealistic expectations or are bothered by a behavior that others can easily ignore.

When analyzing behaviors, keep the following in mind:
1. Define a specific behavior, not general behavior.
2. Evaluate behavioral variables, such as frequency, intensity, duration, and impact.
3. Define parameters of occurrence, such as when, where, and with whom.
4. Determine the time, energy, cost and impact of changing this behavior. Is it worth addressing?
5. Remember, if behavior isn't defined carefully, it will not modify in response to intervention. Careful assessment is prerequisite to intervention; otherwise, no one knows what it is we're trying to change!

✔ **Identify target behaviors for modification.**
Behavior targets should be defined in clear, measurable terms. This will facilitate observation of changes on the part of both the child and teachers. A good test to determine if a behavior is clearly defined is to ask someone else to chart or measure its occurrence. If it is clearly defined, observation data should be in fairly close agreement.

For example, a target behavior of "Kayla to pay attention during math instruction" is too general to measure. It would need to be defined more specifically as "Kayla's behavior will constitute her paying attention during math class if she exhibits the following: looking at her math book or paper, looking at the teacher or board, looking at other students answering or asking questions, or looking at materials being presented." Other behaviors can then be classified as "not paying attention."

It is also important to limit behavioral targets. Choose the most disruptive or those with the most the significant adverse impact on the student or other students in the class. It is not realistic to go from one extreme to the other by implementing a modification program. Steps must be small and minimal so the student's focus is not diluted. The student should have only one or two targets to focus on so she can channel maximum energy toward those behavioral goals. Once accomplished, a new behavioral target can be substituted for one successfully resolved or under control.

✔ **Identify positive reinforcements and incentives.**
There are a variety of reinforcement options to consider when designing behavioral modification programs for children with ADD/ADHD. The most important is that the presentation of the consequence increases or maintains the targeted behavior. When considering positive reinforcements, it is important to consider the following:

- The student will only have access to the reinforcement if it has been earned.
- Reinforcement must be positive for the child (i.e., what he likes rather than what you like).
- Reinforcements increase approximations of the targeted final behavior.
- Reinforcements begin on a continuous immediate schedule to build the incidence of targeted behavior and fade to intermittent as behavior stabilizes.

Some of the major variables to consider in determining reinforcements are listed and explained below and on the following page.

1. *Primary and secondary reinforcements*—Primary reinforcements are usually defined as natural, biological, unlearned consequences, such as edibles (e.g., foods and liquids) or sensory experiences (e.g., listening to music through headphones). Secondary reinforcements are learned or conditioned consequences, such as tangible objects (e.g., stickers, pencils, trinkets, toys), privileges (e.g., first to recess, line leader, computer game time, messenger), and social reinforcement (e.g., smiles, wink, physical proximity, praise). Primary reinforcements should be used when students are learning the new behavioral response because they are more powerful and likely to increase targeted behavior occurrence. They should be paired gradually with

secondary reinforcements, and then secondary used to stabilize the behavior while primary reinforcers stay with new targets.

2. *Token economies*—A token economy would be classified as a generalized secondary reinforcement option. The best analogy would be the monetary system used culturally. The tokens earned can be traded for back-up reinforcers with assigned values, giving the student a choice of options. For example, token points could be traded in for a no homework pass at 100 points, no math homework at 50 points, 30 points for a soda, 25 points for a new pen/pencil, and 15 points for 10 minutes of computer time. Some guidelines for token economy systems are the following:

   • Clearly post and label points to earn specific items.

   • Insure options along a wide continuum for the student who needs more immediate gratification versus one working toward more delayed gratification.

   • Choose tokens that are not easily accessible otherwise so the student can't manipulate the system.

   • Provide a secure place for token storage.

   • Arrange a record-keeping system so students can tally their tokens and concretely see progress toward pay-off opportunities.

3. *Schedules and levels of reinforcement systems*—The schedule of reinforcement and level of rewards controls the timing and delivery of positive incentives for students. Continuous schedules of reinforcement (i.e., every time the behavior occurs it is rewarded) are subject to satiation and need to be modified to an intermittent schedule (i.e., some but not all occurrences of the target behavior are rewarded) as soon as possible to insure maintenance of the targeted behavior. For example, rather than rewarding the student every time he exhibits a target behavior, reward him for some, but not all, occurrences. A ratio schedule can also be used as an intermittent reward system, which would provide the reinforcement based on a time or number interval. The interval can be fixed or variable. The important factor to consider when determining these variables is to insure attainment for the student. If goals are unrealistic and the student never achieves the payoff level, then the system will not increase the likelihood of the targeted behavior. Some guidelines to consider when determining reinforcement schedules are listed on the following page.

- Determine an entry level for the student using behavioral observation data.
- Determine terminal expectations levels for the targeted behavior.
- Determine appropriate rewards and privileges that will be positive and motivating for the specific students.
- Determine the specifics of implementing the system and make sure everyone is clear and consistent (e.g., who charts, when charting occurs, when pay-offs can be requested, etc.).
- Make sure the behavioral expectation is simple, positive, and clear to all involved.

✔ **Identify contingencies or consequences to be used in conjunction with positive incentives.**

Contingency contracts can be used to formalize a behavioral agreement. Specified components would be the targeted behavior at specified performance level, date to be completed, and predetermined reward for the student if contract is met. The student and teacher can sign and date the document together to make it official. The contract focuses the student and teacher on the behavioral goal in a way that is clear, honest, and fair to both parties. This prevents hidden agendas, unrealistic or changing expectations, and an agreed upon reward that is proportional to the targeted goal.

Additional consequences are sometimes imposed to decrease incidence of inappropriate behavior. In conjunction with earning positive reinforcements, consequences can be introduced to focus the student on not receiving the positive reinforcement. Examples include the following:

- *Punishment*—punishment results in decreasing future occurrences of a behavior. A punishment would be a consequence that is introduced immediately following a behavior that reduced the likelihood of the behavior occurring again.
- *Extinction*—extinction involves withholding reinforcement that is maintaining an inappropriate behavior. For example, if rude comments result in teacher attention, then they are ignored so they do not result in attention.

- *Time-out*—time-out stands for "time-out from positive reinforcement." It is actually a punishment because it removes the opportunity to earn positive rewards or reinforcement. Time-out can be exclusionary (removed from opportunity for positive reinforcement) or seclusionary (isolated from the ongoing activity).

✔ **Apply strategies to decrease inappropriate behaviors and increase appropriate behaviors.**
Target behaviors will need to be shaped or gradually approximated through a series of sequenced steps. It is not realistic to expect a student with ADD/ADHD to go from attending for approximately 10 minutes intermittently in math class to sustained attention throughout the entire 45 minutes. Instead, design a gradual sequence of steps to shape the student's behavior that results in him earning the reinforcement.

Summary Comments

Behavioral models to target inappropriate behavior are well researched in the literature. Behavioral modification can be a powerful teaching strategy when used effectively. Once behaviors are clearly defined and justified through careful observation, positive reinforcement techniques should be initiated to increase appropriate desired behavior. Teachers need to understand the variables involved to promote effective behavior management using realistic expectations. Punishment should not be considered unless appropriate behavior replacement techniques have failed.

Children with ADD/ADHD do not want to be bad. They are not trying to push teachers' buttons and disrupt classroom teaching. It is important to understand a behavior's cause and see it as an over-reactive response to stimuli. Help children with ADD/ADHD learn alternative behavioral responses that build positive self-esteem and productive behavior in the classroom. Remember the formula: **SPC—Simple/Specific, Positive, and Clear.**

Questions & Answers

Why do I have to implement a behavior modification program for a child with ADD/ADHD in the classroom; I don't have to do it for other children?

Like children with other disabilities, ADD/ADHD can be a disability requiring adjustments in the environment. We build ramps in buildings to allow people in wheelchairs to enter, we have Braille on elevator buttons for people unable to see, we use special devices like hearing aides, artificial limbs, and wheelchairs. The "special" devices for children with ADD/ADHD are often behavior modification programs, token systems, and reminder charts. The child with ADD/ADHD needs the structure and clear boundaries in order to achieve success.

Dr. Richard Lavoie discusses the difference between what is fair and what is equal. Equal means that everyone gets the same. Fair means that everyone gets what they need. The implementation of a behavior system is often the "fair" thing for a student with ADD/ADHD.

Jack has been diagnosed with ADD/ADHD. He is on medication; however, he continues to be annoying to others, controlling, and in receipt of negative social feedback from both peers and teachers. What can be done to help Jack?

Due to their impulsivity and activity level, children with ADD/ADHD often seek to solve social problems through physical means. They may have difficulty accepting responsibility for their actions and attribute blame to others, often leading to further difficulties with peer relations. In some instances, the child may have a deficit in social skills. Since school is the most significant socialization agent for a child outside the family, teachers can be actively involved in developing positive social skills using training and self-monitoring strategies.

I have heard that children with ADD/ADHD cannot take responsibility for their behavior and always give excuses for their inappropriate behavior. Is this true?

Therapists, educators, and physicians routinely teach children that ADD/ADHD is a challenge, not an excuse. Medication corrects the student's underlying chemical imbalance, giving them a fair chance of facing the challenges of growing up to become productive citizens. Accommodations for the disabled, as mandated by federal and state laws, are not ways of excusing these individuals from meeting society's responsibilities, but rather make it possible for them to compete on a level playing field.

Chapter 8

Educational Intervention for ADD/ADHD

Case Example

Caleb is repeating first grade due to minimal progress. He experienced difficulty in academic, social, emotional, and behavioral areas. His teacher described him as happy and unconcerned about his problems. He is absent-minded, constantly staring off into space and not paying attention. His feelings are easily hurt when he is corrected or reprimanded, but he quickly forgets and commits the same offense for which he was just punished. He does not complete assignments and rarely remembers when he has a project due. He measures low average on intelligence tests, but his actual academic performance is significantly below that level. He is very talkative, mumbling under his breath all the time. Caleb is always the last to finish any paper, and his writing is very slow, labored, and marked by poor spacing, letter formation, and orientation (i.e., letters backwards). He can't sound out words, and his reading is trial and error, with lots of guesses as to what words might be rather than using any logical reasoning to try and figure them out. Spelling is atrocious, with poor sequencing of letters and no knowledge of rule exceptions. Math is a struggle for memorization of basic facts, and timed tests are always failed as Caleb guesses and makes up answers to try and finish first. He wants friends, but he alienates peers by his immature behavior. The school team believes that by repeating first grade, Caleb will have more time to mature, both socially and mentally.

Educators are often perplexed by the child with ADD/ADHD. The child's behavior is often misunderstood and disruptive in the school setting. Teachers, whose primary goal is the education of children, often find the child with ADD/ADHD difficult to teach in a multi-student setting. This leads to frustration for both the teacher and child.

Students with ADD/ADHD who do not receive adequate and appropriate treatment have a greater likelihood of grade retention, dropping out of school, academic underachievement, and social and emotional adjustment difficulties. This is probably because

ADD/ADHD makes children vulnerable to failure in the two most important arenas for developmental mastery—school performance and peer relations. Children with ADD/ADHD are not unable to learn, but they do have difficulty performing in school due to poor organization, impulsivity/hyperactivity, inattention, and distractibility.

ADD/ADHD frequently coexists with other learning, behavioral, emotional, and developmental problems. These include learning disabilities, particularly reading, writing, spelling, math, speech and language disorders, conduct disorder, oppositional defiant disorder, mood disorders, and anxiety disorders. ADD/ADHD also affects memory, especially working memory and organization.

ADD/ADHD occurs across all levels of intelligence: even bright or gifted children with ADD/ADHD may experience school failure. Despite natural ability, their inattentiveness, impulsivity, and hyperactivity can result in failing grades, retention, suspension, and expulsion. Without proper diagnosis, accommodations, and intervention, children with ADD/ADHD are more likely to experience negative consequences.

If ADD/ADHD is left untreated, it can lead to poor self-esteem and social adjustment. Children with ADD/ADHD commonly experience interpersonal difficulties and peer rejection, and have been shown to elicit more negative feedback from teachers. However, teachers do not have to face these challenges alone: they work as part of a team that includes administrators, school psychologists, healthcare professionals, and the parents.

Research has identified effective interventions for addressing the academic, behavioral, and psychological needs of children with ADD/ADHD and their families (Barkley, 1990; DuPaul & Stoner, 1994; Teeter, 1991; Teeter & Semrud-Clikeman, 1995; Weiss & Hechtman, 1993). However, data suggest that children with ADD/ADHD often have high rates of learning problems and under-achievement (Fischer, Barkley, Fletcher, & Smallish, 1990; Semrud-Clikeman, Biederman et al., 1992). Thus, school professionals need to bring research into the classrooms by becoming more knowledgeable about educational "best practices" for children with ADD/ADHD and by coordinating their efforts with team members.

A child with ADD/ADHD can excel to his ultimate potential with educational interventions and classroom accommodations designed to fit the needs of the child. Many of the suggestions listed in this chapter can prove beneficial for all children, not just for the child with ADD/ADHD.

Principles of Program Design

Schools that are most successful in helping students with ADD/ADHD make certain that individual student differences are reflected in the design of their education plans. Teachers and administrators demonstrate a common commitment to working with students with ADD/ADHD. They understand the complexity of the disorder and believe strongly in the services being provided to all children. Personnel in successful schools work together as a team to deal effectively with students with ADD/ADHD by matching techniques and modifications to students' individual potential and methods of learning.

Responsive schools organize their programs and instruction to meet the special needs of all students, including those with ADD/ADHD. In redesigned programs, the entire class participates in a system that does not separate the child with ADD/ADHD from the rest of the group. Programs range from a simple "target behavior of the day" with an immediate reward system to an elaborate system of "levels" in which each level has specific rules and privileges. Schools vary their activities, use cooperative learning and games as part of their strategy, and provide additional training for teachers who need it.

Since students with ADD/ADHD can experience rejection by their fellow students, successful school programs include training in social skills and pairing students with peers without ADD/ADHD. These schools can also serve as partners for parents and develop a common understanding of goals and objectives, as well as a shared plan to carry out objectives and communicate progress and/or problems.

Students with ADD/ADHD and other attention or behavior problems do best in a structured classroom, one where expectations and rules are clearly communicated to them and where academic tasks are carefully designed for manageability and clarity.

Successful schools realize that students with ADD/ADHD are not "problem children," but rather children with a problem. They encourage the school, parents, and teachers to work together with the child with ADD/ADHD in order to help that child develop skills and work habits that he will need to be successful in school and in life.

Improving the quality of the teaching-learning process requires the teacher to make the best possible match between the student's learning preferences, the curriculum to be taught, and the teaching strategy to be used. Teachers should carefully evaluate these three components.

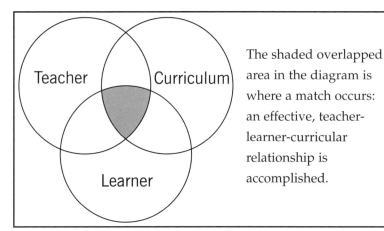

The shaded overlapped area in the diagram is where a match occurs: an effective, teacher-learner-curricular relationship is accomplished.

The acts of teaching and learning (as illustrated in the figure on the left) put the teacher in the role of the decision maker. To accomplish this match effectively, teacher decisions should be made from options available within the instructional variables of setting, content, operations, process, and evaluation.

Setting

- whom to teach
- assessment of student needs, interests, abilities, and styles
- physical setting
- classroom organization
- psychological climate

Content

- what to teach
- quality, quantity
- order, sequence
- materials, equipment
- mode and media

Operations

- thinking and feeling processes
- introversion/extroversion preferences
- tasks and activities to be performed

Process

- teaching strategies to be used
- student roles, teacher roles
- implementation procedures

Evaluation

- giving and receiving feedback
- establishing criteria for successful performance (product and process)
- collecting, analyzing, and utilizing data for future learning

It is important that the teacher assume responsibility for determining strategies to assist students with ADD/ADHD. Too often teachers agree to accommodate the student if told what they need to do. It is the teacher's expertise and experience that should guide those decisions.

One widespread, successful model for daily lesson planning has evolved from Madeline Hunter's (1982) work. Components of this lesson design model include the following:

1. *Anticipatory Set*
   This component captures the student's focus and attention. It is most effective when it does the following:
   a. allows students to remember an experience that will help them acquire new learning
   b. involves active student participation
   c. is relevant

2. *Learning Objective*
   This is a clear statement of what students are expected to accomplish during a learning episode.

3. *Purpose*

   This states why the students should accomplish the learning objective. Whenever possible, it should refer to how the new learning is related to prior and future learning.

4. *Input*

   This is the information and procedures that students will need to accomplish the learning objective. It can and should take on many forms, such as cooperative learning groups, role-playing, small group discussions, etc.

5. *Modeling*

   The teacher must first present models that are accurate, unambiguous, and non-controversial.

6. *Check for Understanding*

   These are strategies teachers use during learning activities to verify that students are accomplishing the learning objective. Checks for comprehension could be accomplished in the form of oral discussion, a written quiz, or other means to verify student learning.

7. *Guided Practice*

   During this time, the student applies new learning in the presence of the teacher, who provides immediate feedback on the accuracy of the learner's practice.

8. *Reflection*

   This is a time when the learner can summarize for himself the perception of what he has learned.

9. *Independent Practice*

   The learner attempts to implement new skills on his/her own to enhance retention.

Additional considerations for daily instructional planning include the following:
- Learning engages the entire person (cognitive, affective, and psychomotor domains).
- The human brain seeks patterns in its search for meaning.
- Emotions are an integral part of learning, retention, and recall.
- Transfer always affects new learning.
- The brain's working memory has a limited capacity.
- Lecture results in the lowest degree of retention.
- Rehearsal is essential for retention.

- The brain is a parallel processor performing many functions simultaneously.
- Each brain is unique.

The teacher's approach should be consistent with the neurology of ADD/ADHD and brain differences that result. (This information was discussed in Chapter 5.) Those principles can be expanded to help the teacher decide on appropriate strategies in the educational setting. To assist in this process, a Report Card (on the next two pages) was developed for the teacher that addresses incorporation of brain-based strategies.

Brain-based Report Card on Teaching Strategies

Instructional Strategy Categories	Not Using	Minimal Use	Doing Well
Attention			
Ability to gain student's attention when appropriate			
Balance of novelty, ritual, and challenge			
Appropriate use of nonverbal gestures for attention			
Use of posters, peripherals, and multi-sensory stimuli			
Offering learner choices for topics and activities			
Use of music, video, guest speakers, computers, etc.			
Physically comfortable environment with choices			
Longer time invested on fewer, more complex topics			
Time flexibility on work activities and projects			
Management and empowerment of learner states			
Motivation			
Use of non-hostile, non-threatening discipline system			
Emphasis on preventative and invisible discipline			
Purposeful and productive activation of emotions			
Create a safe, secure environment without threats			
Immediate and consistent learner feedback			
Continuous daily feedback with de-emphasis on testing			
Student input and dialogue in evaluation process			
Realistic, daily goal setting with student input			
Model joy of learning and excitement for topics			
Relevant, real-life experiences with personal options			

The Source for ADD/ADHD

Brain-based Report Card on Teaching Strategies, *continued*

Instructional Strategy Categories	Not Using	Minimal Use	Doing Well
Movement/Environment			
Consistent alternation of movement and sitting activities			
Exercise opportunities for students available daily			
Water available to students on consistent basis			
Change in location for different activities			
Rhythm and music incorporated into learning			
Students input allowed on room temperature			
Lighting options vary			
Alternative seating options/learning postures are available			
Noise is controlled or monitored			
Classroom is visually organized to facilitate learning			
General Strategies			
Use of natural memory (context, motor, sensory)			
Use of collaborative learning teams			
Use of integrated, multidisciplinary thematic units			
Specific "how-to" strategies are learned and demonstrated			
Maintaining logs or portfolios on student changes over time			
Students have opportunity to explain or defend personal bias			
Teacher-student relationships based on trust			
Use of multiple intelligences in evidence of content mastery			
Students encouraged to show personal relevance			
Students demonstrate mastery of process of learning as well as content			

Suggestions for ideas in the major areas included on the Report Card assessment are discussed in the following section.

Attention: Getting It, Focusing It, Keeping It

Being able to catch and hold a student's interest and attention is not always an easy task. Keeping a student with ADD/ADHD focused and on-task is a monumental challenge to teachers, and one that requires trying a variety of approaches.

Although students with ADD/ADHD are easily distracted, simple methods can help them focus their attention. These include placing students near your desk or in the front row, maintaining eye contact with the students, using gestures to emphasize points, and providing a work area away from distractions. Reduce the amount of materials present during work time by having the student put away unnecessary items. Have a special place for tools, materials, and books.

You can help students shift from one task to another by providing clear and consistent transitions between activities or warning students a few minutes before changing activities. Similarly, when you ask a student with ADD/ADHD a question, begin the question with the child's name and then pause for a few seconds as a signal to the child to pay close attention. Some specific strategies are listed in the following section.

✔ **Ideas to Get Students' Attention**

1. Signal your students using any number of techniques—turning off the lights, flashing the lights, ringing a bell, raising your hand (which signals the children to raise their hands and close their mouths until everyone is quiet), playing a bar of music, etc.

2. Vary tone and/or volume of voice, such as using loud, soft, or whispered directions. For example, a loud command (e.g., "Listen! Ready! Freeze!") could be followed by a few seconds of silence before proceeding in a normal voice to give directions.

3. Maintain eye contact. Students should be facing you when you are speaking, especially while you are giving instructions. Teachers who have students seated with desks in clusters need to work out a structure to have students turn their chairs and bodies around to face the teacher when signaled to do so.

4. Model excitement and enthusiasm about the upcoming lesson.

5. Ask the class an interesting question to generate discussion and interest in the upcoming lesson.

✔ **Ideas to Focus Students' Attention**

1. Employ multisensory strategies when giving directions and presenting lessons.

2. Use visual stimuli. Write key words or draw pictures on the board or overhead projector, use Powerpoint, Hyperstudio, Kids Pix, or other software programs that incorporate graphics.

3. Add color. Use colored chalk to highlight on the chalkboard, and colored pens on the overhead.

4. Use your hands or a colored box to frame the visual material you want students to focus on.

5. Point to written material you want students to focus on. Use a pointer, flashlight, or laser pointer.

6. Incorporate demonstrations and hands-on presentations into your teaching whenever possible.

7. Explain the purpose and relevance to hook students into the lesson.

8. Project your voice and make sure you can be heard clearly by all students. Be aware of competing sounds in your room environment.

✔ **Ideas for Helping Distractible Students**

1. Seat students near you to limit distractions.

2. Make direct eye contact with students.

3. Request that students clear their desks from distractions.

4. Seat the child among attentive, well-focused students.

5. Use physical contact (e.g., hand on shoulder).

6. Incorporate positive reinforcement and behavior modification techniques (e.g., contracts, points, etc.).

7. Praise the student when she is focused with comments such as, "I like the way Cassie is sitting up and looking at me."

8. Use a private signal that you have arranged with the student to help focus attention. For example, when the teacher touches her ear, it is a reminder to "listen."

✔ **Maintaining Attention and Keeping Students Involved**

1. Keep the lesson clear.

2. Present at a brisk pace.

3. Be prepared to reduce off-task behaviors as they occur.

4. Use pictures, diagrams, gestures, manipulatives, and high interest materials.

5. Design activities to be completed in pairs or small groups. Cooperative learning can be an ideal structure for keeping students engaged in an activity.

6. Use higher-level questioning techniques. Ask questions that are open-ended, requiring reasoning and critical thinking.

7. Allow at least five seconds of wait time. Many students need additional time to process a question, gather their thoughts, and formulate an expressive response. Try rephrasing questions to enhance processing.

Motivation, Movement, and the Environment

Because no two children with ADD/ADHD are alike, no single educational setting, practice, or plan will be best for all children. Instead, teachers can help all students by identifying individual strengths and special learning needs and designing a plan for mobilizing those strengths to improve students' academic and social performance.

Recent research suggests that providing more stimulation and variety can improve the performance and behavior of students with ADD/ADHD. You can alter the type of assignment, the activities involved, or even the color of the paper used.

Lessons can be structured individually, competitively, or cooperatively. There is a place for all three structures in the classroom; however, research shows that cooperative learning is the most effective structure. Unfortunately, it is also the one that is used least. Whenever possible, teach lessons using the cooperative structure. Provide many opportunities for students to work with partners or in groups of three or four. The reasons students with attention difficulties, as well as the general student population, gain a great deal from a cooperative learning structure are stated on the following page.

- Students can receive more immediate feedback.
- Students have a shorter wait before being able to share/respond.
- A small group is the best place for learning and practicing social skills.

Even though students with ADD/ADHD may have difficulty staying on task within a group, they are typically better engaged than they would be if working individually or competitively.

A series of learning style adaptations are listed for teachers to consider, not only for the benefit of students with ADD/ADHD, but also for all students.

- Present new information through multisensory instruction. Involve all of the senses, providing auditory, visual, and tactile-kinesthetic input.
- When you need to re-teach information, try it in a variety of different ways.
- For **visual learners**, supply maps, graphs, pictures, and diagrams. Write on overhead/board with colored markers, pens, or chalk.
- Point, highlight, model, and demonstrate.
- Teach through clustering, mind mapping, and other graphic organizers.
- For **global learners** who need to see the whole picture before making sense of the parts, show the end product.
- For **auditory learners**, read aloud; paraphrase; and utilize music, rhythm, melody, discussion, and tapes.
- Have material that students need to learn on tape so they can listen to it. Allow students to bring in small tape recorders to record teacher lectures and supplement note-taking.
- For **tactile/kinesthetic learners**, provide lots of hands-on experiences that promote learning by doing. Use manipulatives for teaching and take time to utilize role-play, dance movement, and acting-out.
- Use computers and games.
- Offer many choices (e.g., book reports, science projects, oral reports).
- Hook the students into the instruction emotionally.
- Let students know why material being presented is important to them.
- Alter the instructional groupings in your class (for example, by interest, skill, or topic).
- Individualize activities and assignments. For example, provide contract packages for students to choose activities from.

- Offer some competitive activities (team games) in class.
- Allow students to use learning aids (tape recorder, reference charts, calculators, typewriter, word processor, spell-checks).
- Use meaning-making strategies (metacognition, reciprocal teaching, think-alouds) in all content areas.
- Teach visualization strategies. Help students develop the strategy of making a detailed mental picture.
- Encourage students to look for or identify patterns in math, literature, poetry, nature, music, dance, etc.
- Use a "discovery" approach as often as possible in teaching. Let students do the experimenting and discover on their own.
- Teach students to explain their reasoning and describe their thinking processes in writing. For example, ask "How did you go about solving the problem?"
- Bring humor into the classroom.
- Consider student interests in planning lessons.
- Teach students to use mnemonics (memory devices or tricks to memorize things). Examples include "Every Good Boy Does Fine" for learning "line notes" on the treble staff; the state of Louisiana looks like a boot; or "Roy G. BIV" for the seven colors in the visible spectrum/rainbow (red, orange, yellow, green, blue, indigo, violet).
- Allow for physical needs. When students are physically uncomfortable (need to go to bathroom or are hungry, hot, or thirsty), they will not be able to focus on instruction. Many teachers allow students to bring water bottles to class, especially on hot days. Teachers can also keep crackers or other snack foods available for hungry children.

General Strategies

✔ **Organization and Study Skills**
Students with ADD/ADHD often have significant challenges with organization and study skills. This is, in fact, one of the key characteristics of the disorder. These students need direct assistance, structuring, and training in how to effectively do the following:

- Organize their materials.
- Organize their workspace.

- Record their assignments.
- Make lists.
- Prioritize activities.
- Plan for short term-assignments.
- Break down long-term assignments.
- Know the standards of acceptable work for each class.
- Read and use a calendar.
- Read a clock and follow a schedule.
- Know what to take home and leave home.
- Know when and where to turn in assignments.
- Know what to do when seatwork is completed.
- Know what materials are needed and expected for each class.

✔ **Tips for Giving Directions**

It is important to spend time making sure students with ADD/ADHD clearly understand directions . It is not unusual to sabotage chances for success in the student with ADD/ADHD before the assignment even begins due to confusion in what the parameters of the assignment are. The following suggestions will assist students in successfully following directions:

1. Wait until the entire class is quiet before giving directions.
2. Wait until you have everyone's attention. You may need to walk over and touch or physically cue certain students to achieve their focus.
3. Explain directions clearly and concisely.
4. Face students when you talk.
5. Use multisensory instructions. Provide visual and verbal instructions.
6. Model what to do. Show the class.
7. Don't overwhelm students with too much at one time.
8. Have students record on a calendar when the assignment is due.
9. Check for understanding.
10. Have individual students repeat or rephrase directions back to you to check for understanding.
11. Make sure to give complete directions, including what you expect students to do once the task is finished.

✔ **Additional Strategy Ideas**

Students with ADD /ADHD may need more help than their peers in learning strategies to help them study and organize their work efficiently. Assistance in these areas might include focusing on listening skills, outlining structure, task structuring, and notebook organization. Teach students techniques for taking notes from both lectures and textbooks. Some teachers have found it helpful to give their students an outline for their notes and to list the main ideas or concepts in advance.

Teachers can break down assignments into smaller, less complex units and build in reinforcement as the student finishes each part. Students with ADD/ADHD may need more time (especially on tests) than other students. You can give a student confidence by starting each assignment with a few questions or activities you know the student can successfully accomplish.

Some teachers have found that pairing a student with ADD/ADHD with another student or dividing the class into cooperative groups can be an effective way to encourage the student to concentrate on the work.

Students may need both verbal and visual directions. Provide the child with a model of what he or she should be doing. Periodically remind the student of the assignment and check on progress.

Communication with parents is essential when working with children with ADD/ADHD. A simple way to improve communication is to use a checklist system for parents that records when a student achieves a goal or objective, such as arriving on time, being prepared, and completing classroom work. For each subject, the child should write down the homework assignment and then show it to the teacher so that it can be checked for correctness. At the end of the class, repeat the homework assignment out loud as a reminder. Parents can then use the checklist to ensure that the student with ADD/ADHD completes assigned homework.

Educational Accommodations for the Student with ADD/ADHD

The focus prior to this point has been on options available to the teacher. Decisions must be agreed upon that accommodate a student with ADD/ADHD so she can experience success in the educational setting. The focus at some point needs to shift to the child. The school team and parents need to determine what the special needs of the student with ADD/ADHD are so that everyone involved can be consistent in implementing strategies. A guide to determine necessary accommodations is provided on the following pages. This form allows the educational team to focus on the child's special needs, while providing a format to share impressions with other professionals and the parents.

Accommodation Plan

Name:	Date:
School:	Completed by:

Instructions: Consider the student's area of difficulty. Check (✔) which accommodations are appropriate to meet the student's needs.

1. Attention

	Seat student in a quiet area.
	Seat student near a study buddy.
	Increase distance between desks.
	Seat away from distracting stimuli.
	Allow student extra time to complete assigned work.
	Shorten assignments/work periods.
	Break assignments into smaller parts.
	Require fewer responses.
	Reduce homework assignments.
	Pair with other students to check work.
	Cue student to stay on task, e.g., private signal.
	Other:

2. Impulsiveness

	Ignore minor, inappropriate behavior.
	Increase immediacy of rewards or consequences.
	Supervise/Structure during transition periods.
	Acknowledge good behavior of student or others.
	Seat student near role model or teacher.
	Establish positive behavior contracts.
	Instruct student in self-monitoring behavior, e.g., hand raising.
	Implement behavior management system.
	Other:

3. Motor Activity

	Allow student to stand at times while working.
	Provide opportunities for breaks between assignments.
	Remind student to check over work.
	Provide student extra time to complete assignments.
	Other:

4. Organization and Planning

	Provide rules for organization.
	Encourage student to have notebook with dividers and folders for work.
	Provide a homework assignment book and/or checklist.
	Send daily/weekly progress reports home.
	Allow student to have an extra set of books at home.
	Provide peer assistance with organization.

4. Organization and Planning, *continued*

	Give assignments one at a time.
	Establish short-term goals in completing assignments.
	Do not penalize for handwriting if student has visual motor or organizational deficits.
	Encourage student to learn keyboarding skills.
	Allow tape recording.
	Use visual aids in lesson presentation.
	Other:

5. Compliance

	Praise compliant behavior.
	Post class rules.
	Provide immediate feedback about behavior.
	Ignore minor inappropriate behavior.
	Use prudent reprimands for misbehavior, e.g., avoid lecturing.
	Implement behavior management system.
	Assist student in self-monitoring, e.g., following directions, raising hand to talk.
	Other:

6. Mood

	Provide reassurance and encouragement.
	Compliment positive behavior and work.
	Review instructions for new assignments to make sure student understands.
	Provide opportunities for student to display leadership role in class.
	Focus on student's accomplishments.
	Conference frequently with student and parents to learn more about the student's interests and achievements.
	Send positive notes home.
	Encourage social interactions with others.
	Teach appropriate social skills.
	Other:

7. Socialization

	Praise appropriate social behavior.
	Set up social behavior goals with student and implement an incentive program.
	Prompt appropriate social behavior either verbally or with a private signal.
	Encourage student to observe classmate who exhibits appropriate social skills.
	Encourage cooperative learning tasks.
	Provide small group social skills training in class.
	Other:

8. Other Accommodations

	Schedule regular parent-teacher conferences.
	Assist physician in monitoring behavior and attention if medication is prescribed.
	Other:

Summary

I have come to a frightening conclusion
That I am the decisive element in the classroom.
It's my personal approach that creates the climate.
It's my daily mood that makes the weather.

As a teacher, I possess a tremendous power
To make a child's life miserable or joyous.
I can be a tool of torture
Or an instrument of inspiration.
I can humiliate or humor, hurt or heal.

In all situations, it is my response
That decides whether a crisis will be
Escalated or de-escalated
And a child humanized or dehumanized
                                        —Haim Ginott

Ginott, H., *Teacher and Child*, The McMillian Co., New York, 1972

Questions & Answers

*When should new information be introduced in the classroom
to ensure better retention?*

For students to remember new information, it must be repeated. Monday, Tuesday, and perhaps Wednesday are good days for introducing information. Thursday and Friday are less desirable days because students will not have enough time to activate long-term memory prior to the weekend.

Because most people remember beginnings and endings better than middle sections, important information should be presented at the beginning of class. Pre-exposure can also be a powerful way to help students make connections to new material. Discussion prior to presentation of content is also helpful.

Chapter 5 discussed neurology and its impact on learning. How can I make my classroom more brain compatible?

There are many options. You can use multiple intelligences, learning styles, or differentiated teaching strategies. These will make your teaching more brain compatible. Decide which of these fit your teaching style.

Create colorful posters with positive affirmations. Replace white chalk with colored chalk to make using the chalkboard more fun and appealing. Have students work in teams and assess their skills in group settings. Teach in a multi-modal fashion, making sure every lesson contains a visual, auditory, and kinesthetic component.

What advice can be given to teachers as they prepare to educate students with ADD/ADHD?

Some of the best advice offered to teachers comes from adults with ADD/ADHD who share some of their experiences. The following is one example: "I guess I would tell teachers that there are a thousand roads to roam. Not everyone is going to choose the same path. Everybody has different ways of assimilating data-different filters, different life experiences that affect how they look at things and process information. To be fair, teachers need to first evaluate if some other method of learning is available to help one child or another to do what they have to do. For me to do my best, put me in a group of three or four people. I get the most from a group structure where there is a lot of verbal interaction."

I just finished my first year of teaching and was amazed at the number of students that had different learning styles, especially students with ADD/ADHD. The teacher in the room next to mine stated that I will encounter these types of needs every year. What are some of the more common challenges I will have in my classroom and ways to effectively handle them?

Some of the more common challenges a teacher is likely to encounter in the education setting are listed on the following page, followed by effective guidelines for intervention.

Common Student Issues and Concerns
- determining who is ADD/ADHD
- dealing with off-task behaviors
- managing disruptive behaviors
- managing inappropriate behaviors
- dealing with an inability to focus
- handling low student self-esteem
- communicating with everyone working with the child
- addressing academic difficulties
- addressing social/peer problems
- dealing with poor study skills
- handling poor test-taking ability
- dealing with poor organization skills

Possible Intervention Ideas
- Give clear and concise directions.
- Make frequent contacts with the student.
- Use a multisensory approach to instruction.
- Provide students with options to break up long periods of sitting.
- Communicate regularly with parents.
- Surround the student with good role models.
- Avoid changes in schedule.
- Maintain consistency.
- Provide positive reinforcement.
- Use technology.
- Give praise immediately.
- Design a motivating classroom environment.
- Make sure classroom rules are clearly defined and consistently enforced.

Chapter 9

Home Intervention for ADD/ADHD

Case Example

What have we done to make our child this way? Are we terrible parents? I feel guilty when the school says he can do better than he is; they make it sound like it is our fault. The teacher hints that we don't discipline him and that we let him get his way. They ought to live with us for one weekend or evening! We try so hard with this child and give him so much more time than the other kids, and for what? Only to be criticized more? Sometimes I get so angry and his father just gives up; then we both feel guilty and decide to start all over again. It's a never ending battlefield to get him to do anything at home. We struggle through hours of homework every night. He can't ever find anything to get ready in the morning. He forgets to tell us about meetings, papers to sign, materials he needs for projects—and then he and the teachers are mad at us for not complying. We can't win! And we're burned out trying. We have to get some help from somewhere!

It's not easy to be a parent these days. When the system at large fails, the blame tends to fall on the parents in the home setting. Parents are willing to travel extensive distances to have their child evaluated by "specialists" and "experts" who all say different things and make conflicting recommendations. It is very difficult for a parent to sort out ADD/ADHD variables when the professionals don't agree on many factors in the disorder area.

Parenting a child with ADD/ADHD or any disability can be overwhelming at times. All parents sometimes feel anger, fear, grief, frustration, and fatigue while struggling to help their child. But parents shouldn't blame themselves for the problems associated with the disorder. ADD/ADHD is a brain-based disorder, and it is not caused by poor parenting or a chaotic environment.

Although life with a child who has ADD/ADHD can be challenging, it is important to remember that children with the disorder can and do succeed. A parent can play a very valuable role in creating home and school environments that improve the child's chances for success. The earlier the child's problems are addressed, the better the chances of preventing school and social failure. Early intervention is the key to maximizing positive outcomes for the child with ADD/ADHD.

This chapter will address some of the more challenging aspects of dealing with ADD/ADHD in the home setting. While every child is an individual, the general strategies suggested are based on principles that can be effective with a wide variety of individuals.

Effective Parenting Strategies

While no treatment can "cure" ADD/ADHD, the following ideas can help a parent be as effective as possible.

1. Look for current, scientifically supported information about ADD/ADHD. A routine task for parents is educating other adults in the child's life about the disorder. Relatives, teachers, and caretakers need to understand that ADD/ADHD is neurobiological and is not the result of too much sugar or too little discipline. They also need to know how they can help the child meet expectations for effective, productive performance and behavior.

2. Secure a professional evaluation and treatment recommendations. A thorough assessment of a child's strengths and weaknesses will help parents and educators develop an appropriate and effective intervention plan that is realistic for the specific child with ADD/ADHD.

3. Become the child's best advocate. The more knowledge parents have about rights for the disabled under the two education laws [Section 504 of the Rehabilitation Act and Individuals with Disabilities Education Act (IDEA)] the better the chances to maximize positive outcomes.

4. Seek parent training from a qualified professional who is experienced in ADD/ADHD. Effective parent training will introduce strategies to change behavior and improve relationships with a child. Parent training should teach parents how to accomplish some of the following:
   • Provide clear, consistent expectations, directions, and limits.
   • Set up an effective discipline system.
   • Create a behavior modification plan to change the most problematic behaviors.
   • Assist the child with social issues.

- Identify the child's strengths and build on them to achieve a sense of pride and accomplishment for the child.
- Set aside a daily "special time" for the child.

5. Find a parental support network. Parents can provide excellent information and support to each other. Parenting a child with a disability is not an easy task, and the constant demands can take a toll on even the very best parents. Seek marital counseling, if necessary, or individual counseling if parents begin feeling overwhelmed or defeated.

6. Tell the child that she is loved and supported unconditionally. The child with ADD/ADHD needs to know that parents are willing to weather the storms with her and that she won't be abandoned when things aren't going well.

Developing Self-Esteem in the Child with ADD/ADHD

Most parents are aware that their child's feelings of self-worth are linked with their success socially and academically. What parents don't always realize is how fragile a child's self-esteem can be and how easily it can be damaged. Research shows that children with disabilities are more likely to suffer from a lack of self-esteem than their peers. Dr. Robert Brooks has compiled a list of suggestions for parents to assist in developing positive feelings of self-worth in their children.

✔ **Help a child feel special and appreciated.**
   Research indicates that one of the main factors that contributes to a child developing hope and becoming resilient toward difficulties is the presence of at least one adult who helps the child feel special and appreciated—an adult who does not ignore a child's problems, but focuses energy on a child's strengths. One idea for parents to achieve this is to set aside "special time" during the week to spend with each child in the household. Let the child know that he is the priority during that time. Don't answer the phone if it rings. Focus on things the child enjoys so that he has an opportunity to relax and demonstrate individual strengths.

✔ **Help a child develop problem-solving and decision-making skills.**
High self-esteem is associated with problem-solving skills. For example, if a child is having difficulty with a friend, ask him to think about a couple of ways of resolving the situation. Don't become upset or worried if the child can't think of any solutions immediately; help him reflect upon possible solutions. Role-playing might also work well to assist a child with generating solutions or possible steps to resolve a problem.

✔ **Avoid judgmental comments: frame comments to be positive and constructive.**
Children are less defensive when a problem is approached with strategies rather than criticism of the action or motivation taken. Identifying deficits isn't always the best way to change a child's mind or introduce a better strategy. For example, a comment that often sounds accusatory is, "Try harder and put in more effort." Many children do try hard but still encounter difficulty. Instead say, "We need to figure a better way for you to learn."

✔ **Be an empathetic parent.**
Many well-intentioned parents become frustrated and blurt out comments like, " Why don't you listen to me?" or "Why don't you use your brain?" If a child is having difficulty learning, it is best to be empathetic and tell him that you recognize he is having difficulty and want to help. The focus should be on the problem to be solved and the energy spent thinking of solutions.

✔ **Provide choices for a child.**
Choices help minimize power struggles. For example, ask a child if he would like to be reminded 5 or 10 minutes before bedtime to begin getting ready. This allows the child to assume some control of the situation and have some say in home procedures.

✔ **Highlight the individual child's strengths.**
Many children with ADD/ADHD view themselves in a negative way, especially in regard to school. Make a list of your child's areas of competence or strength. Find ways to reinforce those strengths and opportunities for the child to display them. For example, if the child is a wonderful artist, display his artwork. Don't compare siblings and list strengths of all

children in a family together: the child with ADD/ADHD is likely to come up short in comparison. Let each child stand alone.

✔ **Provide opportunities for children to help.**
Children seem to have an inborn need to help others. Providing opportunities for children to help is a way of letting them realize they have skills to offer the world. Involving a child in charitable work is one example. Helping others can boost self-esteem

If your child has ADD/ADHD, demystify the nature of the disability and help him understand the disorder. Many children have fantasies and misconceptions about their problems that add to their distress. One child with ADD/ADHD thought he was born with only half a brain! Having realistic information provides a child with a sense of control, understanding, and reassurance that things can be done to help the situation.

Dealing with Everyday Issues

Parents must be effective managers to successfully parent a child with ADD/ADHD. A child with the disorder has poor self-regulation, so parental interactions with the child need to be consistent, predictable, and sympathetic in understanding the everyday difficulties this child experiences. The following guidelines are essential in approaching some of the behavioral challenges.

1. **Education**
   Parents must become educated consumers. They need to thoroughly understand the ADD/ADHD disorder, including developmental, academic, behavioral, and emotional issues.

2. **Incompetence vs. Noncompliance**
   Parents need to develop an understanding of incompetence (non-purposeful problems that result from the child's inconsistent application of skills leading to performance and behavioral deficits) and noncompliance (purposeful problems that occur when children do not want to do as they are asked or directed). This concept was discussed in detail in Chapter 7 on Behavioral Intervention. ADD/ADHD is primarily a disorder of incompetence; however, since at least 50% of children with ADD/ ADHD also experience other disruptive, noncompliant problems, parents must develop a system to differentiate between these two issues and have a set of interventions for both.

3. **Positive Directions**

   Parents should focus on telling children what to do rather than what not to do. Another way to think about this idea is to give children a direction to get them started, not tell them what to stop. This provides an effective, positive direction for the population with ADD/ADHD. Many directions are orders to stop doing something or to not do something at tall. Parents should consciously work on rewording directions in a positive way to help direct a child with ADD/ADHD into a productive behavior.

   > Here are some requests to practice. Reword the following in a positive manner:
   > - Don't stand up when you slide.
   > - Don't stand in the swing.
   > - Don't dump the puzzle pieces on the floor.
   > - Don't hit Tom.
   > - Don't tear the book.
   > - Don't shout.
   > - Don't rock on your chair.
   >
   > How did you do? Here are a few of our suggestions.
   > - Don't stand up when you slide. — *Please sit down when you slide.*
   > - Don't stand in the swing — *Please sit down when you swing.*
   > - Don't dump the puzzle pieces on the floor. — *Please put the puzzle pieces on the table.*
   > - Don't hit Tom. — *Please tell Tom why you are angry with him.*
   > - Don't tear the book. — *The book didn't do anything wrong. Let's just put the book away.*
   > - Don't shout. — *I can hear and we are inside. Let's just talk about this.*
   > - Don't rock on your chair. — *Please keep all the legs of the chair on the floor.*

4. **Rewards**

   Remember that children with ADD/ADHD need more frequent, predictable, and consistent rewards. Both social rewards (praise) and tangible rewards (toys, treats, privileges) must be provided at a higher rate when the child is compliant or succeeds. Remember, it is likely that the child receives less positive reinforcement than siblings. Make an effort to keep the scales balanced. To achieve this, a few suggestions are offered on the following page.

✔ **Timing.** Consequences (both rewards and punishment) must be provided quickly and consistently for them to be meaningful or effective.

✔ **Response Cost.** A modified response cost program (you can lose what you earn) must be utilized with this child at home. This system can provide a child with ADD/ADHD with all the reinforcers at the beginning of the day, and the child must work throughout the day to keep them. Another variation would be to start the child with a blank slate and allow the child to earn at least three to five times the amount of rewards for good behavior versus what she loses for negative behavior (e.g., earn five chips for doing something right, lose one chip for doing something wrong).

5. **Planning**

   Schedule your child's day with an understanding of the positive and negative forces that affect your child with ADD/ADHD. Avoid placing the child in situations in which there is an increased likelihood that temperamental problems will result in difficulty.

6. **Take Care of Yourself**

   Families with children who have ADD/ADHD are likely to experience greater stress, more marital disharmony, and potentially more severe emotional problems that escalate and resolve around the child's behavior. It is important to understand the impact this child may have on a family and deal with the problems in a positive, preventative way rather than a frustrated, angry, and negative way when everyone has reached the end of their patience and tolerance.

7. **Take Care of Your Child**

   Remember that the relationship with a child who has ADD/ADHD is likely to be strained. Take time to foster a positive relationship. Find enjoyable activities and engage in them as often as possible. Outdoor activities with opportunities for movement, running, etc. give the child with ADD/ADHD a chance to run off energy in a constructive way while engaging in relationship-building activities with parents and siblings.

Dealing with the Homework Issue

The struggle to focus a child with ADD/ADHD at home on work that wasn't finished at school can be a nightmare for parents. It is one variable that can ruin everyone's evening by turning the time after dinner into a battle zone of the parents versus the child. Do the following problems sound familiar? They are common homework problems reported by parents of children with ADD/ADHD:

- didn't write down the homework assignment
- wrote down the wrong assignment
- forgot to bring the assignment book home
- forgot the book or materials needed to complete the homework
- taking hours to complete what should take minutes
- arguing about when and where to do homework
- lying about having the homework finished
- requiring constant supervision to stay focused
- needing constant help
- not asking to have homework papers signed
- leaving completed homework at home and forgetting to take it back to school

Parents of children with ADD/ADHD experience a variety of emotions in regard to homework—some positive but most negative. Frustration, annoyance, boredom, confusion, and even anger are among the many negative emotions parents, and their children with ADD/ADHD express when it comes to homework. However, the child's teacher constantly reminds parents that homework is an important component of the school experience. Completing homework successfully teaches students to organize their time, independently structure themselves productively, etc.

Homework continues to be an institution in the educational system. Even in well-functioning families under ideal circumstances, homework can be one of the most volatile parent-child crisis buttons. Parents are unsure as to the best time, place, routine, or system a child should use to complete homework. Many children rebel and parents feel overwhelmed by the pressure of meeting the children's school demands. It is not surprising that parents complain about homework almost as much as their children do.

Homework hassles are not unique to children with ADD/ADHD. Most children forget some assignments, lose homework, require assistance, or make mistakes at some point. Some children have difficulty learning essential skills that enable them to complete homework independently. Some have trouble understanding assignments or writing them down. Some may be confused or overwhelmed with long-term projects. Everyone rushes through assignments at some time.

For children with ADD/ADHD, the challenges of homework are added to existing classroom difficulties. It is not uncommon for these children to bring incomplete classwork home that is added to homework assignments. This results in the prospect of hours and hours of schoolwork at home, often with minimal benefit.

A child's ability to be successful with homework begins with the value parents place on it. Success requires helping a child develop essential homework skills, creating a working alliance with the child and her teachers, and developing strategies to address common homework problems. We've identified five common homework problems that parents of children with ADD/ADHD typically have to deal with.

✔ *The child won't do homework without the parent.*
An important aspect of parenting is to ask about homework and help children successfully complete it. At the elementary school age level, children won't have strategies developed to independently complete homework. Parents should try to develop a structure for homework completion by establishing an agreed upon time, place, and system for completing and monitoring homework each day. The parent involvement should gradually fade so the child learns to complete homework independently, but the parent should always be available for assistance and feedback. Don't correct every wrong answer or complete problems that the child isn't able to do. It isn't the parents' homework, it is the child's and should reflect the child's ability level.

✔ *The child repeatedly makes excuses to avoid doing homework.*
Parents should stay involved with their child's education and study habits to recognize when a pattern has changed and homework habits reflect legitimate struggle versus the usual avoidance excuses. Sometimes "It's too hard" or "I don't understand it" are honest statements. Other times they reflect attempts by a child to avoid working independently. Children

am really impressed: you normally take so long, but you finished in just 30 minutes."

4. Implement a self-monitoring system. The child could wear headphones and listen for a periodic beep that occurs approximately every 30 to 60 seconds. At the beep, the child marks a sheet to indicate whether he was on task or off task. Although this sounds distracting, it can work well to train some children with ADD/ADHD to re-focus independently.

With patience, planning, and creativity, parents can help children with ADD/ADHD experience success with homework.

Dealing with Behavior Issues

A parent or educator who is trying to improve a child's behavior should keep in mind certain basic principles, including the following:

1. Encourage children with ADD/ADHD to take responsibility for their behavior. We can't control others; we can only influence others to want to change their behavior.

2. Establish an atmosphere of mutual respect between parents and the child with ADD/ADHD. Children respond more positively when adults are consistent, honest, open, and supportive.

3. Determine the behavior or events that take place before and after unwanted or undesirable behaviors. It is important to identify the things in the environment that set off or positively reinforce the child's inappropriate behavior. Sometimes the child gets positive reinforcement from the sense of control he feels or the attention he gets from the reaction to his misbehavior. It may be a useful tool for adults to change inappropriate behavior by changing the schedule, modifying events, or avoiding settings that trigger or reinforce inappropriate behavior.

4. Explain expected behaviors and consequences to the child. Parents and teachers should be clear about the kind of behavior desired and the consequences that will follow if the behavior doesn't meet expectations. Remember, **Simple, Positive, and Clear—SPC**! (See Chapter 8.)

5. Establish consequences that are natural and/or logical, and apply the consequences objectively (without anger). If the consequence for hitting a peer is to sit and think for five minutes, then don't also yell or spank the child. This destroys the effect of teaching an appropriate behavior.

6. Give positive reinforcement for appropriate behavior. It is important to make positive reinforcement a natural social reward.

7. Apply consequences or positive reinforcement immediately following the target behaviors. For learning to be effective, a child with ADD/ADHD must be able to clearly relate the consequence or reinforcement to the target behavior.

8. Select only one or two behaviors to modify or teach at a time. Don't try to resolve all issues at once. If too many behaviors are targeted at once, a child with ADD/ADHD will only become confused and may not learn any of the behaviors.

9. Be consistent. It is important for both parents and teachers to be consistent in implementing a child's behavioral program. It's also important for teachers and parents to cooperate in developing the program. Frequent communication between parents and teachers will ensure that the same behavior is expected in all settings and that a misbehavior will result in similar consequences at school and at home.

Shaping Behavior

Sometimes a parent must work to gradually shape a behavior; it is not realistic to expect a child to progress from one extreme to the other without some successive steps in between. Since difficulties with homework were addressed extensively within this chapter, an example of shaping behavior with the homework issue is included in the chart on the following page.

Shaping Behavior

Successive Approximation

Goal: To complete homework assignments independently

This means the child must know the correct assignments and have the right books.

The child will move from Point A to Point B by mastering one step at a time. Each step represents growth and progress toward achieving these goals.

A. Beginning Point: No Homework Done

1. Parents get child started; supervise whole time.
2. Parents get child started; monitor occasionally. Use refocusing prompts as necessary. For example, "You're getting sidetracked."
3. Parents get child started; child finishes.
4. Parent sets timer; child starts homework by self; if child doesn't start, parents prompt after 15 min.; child finishes.
5. Child starts and finishes homework by self; no intervention by parents.

B. Target Behavior: Completes Homework Independently

A. Beginning Point: Doesn't Know Assignments/Doesn't Bring Books Home

1. Child doesn't write down homework assignments; tells parents he doesn't have homework or that it is completed, even if not true.
2. Child forgets to write down assignments most of the time. Parents ask teacher to write down assignments for a week at a time; keep extra set of books at home.
3. Child makes effort to write down assignments but often forgets. Parents ask teachers for homework assignment pattern (e.g., Algebra homework four nights a week, tests every two weeks); get phone number for friend in each class to check assignments when child forgets to write them down.
4. Child remembers to write down assignments sometimes; early afternoon or evening, parents ask if he knows homework assignments; if he forgot, take or send the child back to school to get books and assignments or remind him to call a friend to get assignments.
5. Child remembers right assignments and books most of time; takes responsibility for calling a friend if needed.
6. Child writes down assignments; brings home right books; parents don't need to monitor.

B. Target Behavior: Knows Assignments/Has Books

Summary

This chapter is intended to address some of the main issues that parents of a child with ADD/ADHD face in the home setting. A child's home represents his comfort zone: this is where he freely vents frustration, anger, confusion, and other emotional responses triggered by dealing with ADD/ADHD on a daily basis. Parents bear the brunt of the child's reactions and experience their own frustration of not being able to "fix" things for the child. Parents are also frequently challenged by education professionals to provide answers to dilemmas that they are experiencing in the school setting that they can't cope with or figure out how to circumvent. Every possible scenario has not been addressed. The intention was to provide some global strategies to help parents feel more comfortable facing the challenges presented in the home environment. Certainly additional strategies and suggestions that could be helpful to parents are included throughout the entire book!

Questions & Answers

What are some tips for dealing with siblings of children with ADD/ADHD?

Provide information about ADD/ADHD to all family members. Involve all family members in the interventions. Be aware of sibling anger, jealousy, guilt, and hostility. Remember that siblings can experience the same stages of acceptance as parents. In coming to terms with accepting ADD/ADHD families may experience anger, guilt, shame, and grief. Let each child know that it is acceptable to discuss what she is thinking and feeling. Answer questions about ADD/ADHD factually. Pay positive attention to all family members: remember, spouses and family members without ADD/ADHD need positive feedback too. If needed, seek professional counseling to improve family functioning and communication.

My seven-year-old daughter dawdles when getting ready for school or bed, or when asked to "pick up" her room. Is there any way I can help her to speed up?

To speed up your daughter's slow behavior, try a method called "racing the timer." Set a kitchen timer for a short period of time and reward her if she completes a task before the timer rings. For example, the next time you announce that it's bedtime, set the timer for 15 minutes. Tell her that she gets a bedtime story and a point on the point-reward chart if she beats the timer. To beat the timer she must put on her pajamas, brush her teeth, and be in bed before the timer rings. Don't nag her to hurry and don't scold her if she loses the race; however, when she beats the timer, give her praise, a point on the chart, and a bedtime story!

Are there more ways to use timers to help children?

There are several ways that timers can help improve behavior. Parents can give a time-out to a child that is involved in unacceptable behavior. A timer can also help children to take turns, especially when more than one child wants to play with the same toy. Timers are "parent savers" because they are easy to use, effective in changing behavior, and save "wear and tear" on parents. Timers are also "child savers" because they save children from listening to nagging and lecturing by parents.

My neighbors tell me that they restrict or "ground" their thirteen-year-old son for two or three weeks when he breaks rules. Is this an appropriate method of discipline for my adolescent?

When used correctly, grounding can help preadolescents and teenagers improve their behavior. If you use grounding, be sure you follow two rules: tell your child in advance which misbehaviors will cause "grounding" and keep the duration of grounding short—usually not more than a weekend or one week. Grounding a teenager for a period of two or three weeks is not an effective method for improving behavior.

How can I make my child behave?

- Provide clear, consistent expectations, directions and limits. Children with ADD/ADHD need to know exactly what others expect from them. They do not perform well in ambiguous situations that require determining "shades of gray" or "reading between the lines."
- Set up an effective discipline system. Parents may need to learn proactive discipline methods that teach and reward appropriate behavior and respond to misbehavior with alternatives such as "time-out," natural consequences, and loss of privileges.

- Create a behavior modification plan to change the most problematic behaviors. Behavior charts and other behavior modification techniques will help you focus on and address problems in systematic, effective ways. You will learn to use behavior modification principles to reinforce positive behaviors and to eliminate or reduce negative behaviors that create problems for your child.

- Assist your child with social issues. Children with ADD/ADHD may be rejected by peers because of hyperactive, impulsive, or aggressive behavior. Parent training can help you assist your child in making friends and learning to work cooperatively with others.

- Identify your child's strengths in areas such as art, computers, mechanical ability, etc. and build on these strengths so that your child has a sense of pride and accomplishment.

- Set aside a daily "special time" for your child. Constant negative feedback can erode a child's self-esteem, while a daily dose of TLC— whether a special outing or just time spent in positive interaction— can help fortify your child against assaults to self-worth.

- Seek support for yourself. Parents can give each other information as well as support. Since ADD/ADHD is highly hereditary, many parents of children with ADD/ADHD discover when their child is diagnosed that they too have this disorder. Parents with ADD/ADHD may need the same types of evaluation and treatment that they seek for their children.

How can I help my child make friends?

Almost any program teaching social behaviors involves some form of modeling—that is, demonstrating appropriate behavior so that the child learns by imitation. Role-modeling includes using forceful and interesting verbal cues when speaking, reinforcing good behaviors, offering greetings at the door, and showing appropriate smiles and gestures. For younger children, puppets can be appropriate models. A key part of modeling involves the use of good affective skills and body language. Children with ADD/ADHD may have problems understanding facial expressions. If they are taught how to read the emotions behind such facial expressions, their understanding of social interaction may improve. The child with ADD/ADHD will benefit from immediate feedback (is the parent/teacher angry, pleased, etc.?). Strong affective gestures (winks, thumbs up, frowns, etc.) also communicate effectively to the child. The parent who uses direct, encouraging praise will promote good social response. Encouraging praise places the value on the child's effort, not the quality of outcomes. For example, "I bet you really worked hard on that one." The praise does not judge quality, but it specifically states that the child did well. Do not focus on what the child can't do, but instead focus on the child's strengths and abilities.

> *I'm afraid if I advocate for my child, the school will consider me a troublemaker. Is advocating worth the risk?*

Your child must continue to stay the focus of all your decisions. It is not about who is right or wrong—the school, the physician, or the parent. It IS about what is best for your child. Your child has been diagnosed with ADD/ADHD. If he is to experience success in and/or out of school, all adults having contact with him must communicate and work together. See Chapter 10 for more information.

> *How can I prepare for an evaluation to make sure I ask the right questions and that the professional conducting the evaluation is knowledgeable about ADD/ADHD?*

Questions to ask the professional who may do the assessment:
• How do you diagnose ADD/ADHD?
• Which types of tests or measurements do you use? Do you use the DSM-IV or other reference(s)?
• How do you determine the presenting symptoms and that they exist in at least two settings?
• How long will the assessment take?
• Do other professionals assist in the assessment process?
• What age range do you assess?
• Are you knowledgeable about special services provided at public schools for children and adolescents with ADD/ADHD?
• How long have you been doing assessments for ADD/ADHD?
• If you confirm an ADD/ADHD diagnosis, would you be willing to write a letter to the school or speak to a school official?
• What is your work experience in ADD/ADHD?

- What type of written feedback will I receive when the assessment is completed?
- (If a Clinical Psychologist) Do you work with a specific physician if medication will be involved?

Questions to ask the professional who may do treatment:
- How is medication used in your practice?
- If medication is prescribed, what might be some of the side effects?
- What other therapy in addition to medication might you suggest?
- Is counseling part of the treatment plan?
- If I don't want to put my child on medication, would you attempt to find other possible solutions?
- What are some typical results you have had with your clients? Could you arrange for me to speak with some of them?
- What are your fees? Do you have a sliding scale?
- What can I do at home to help my child?

Review questions for the parent:
- Was this professional easy to talk to?
- Were all of my questions answered satisfactorily?

Chapter 10

Putting It All Together

Case Example

My role at the staffing was to facilitate the discussion and educational plan for an elementary-aged-girl with ADD/ADHD. The conference room had a full representation of various professionals— school psychologist, social worker, speech-language pathologist, occupational therapist, physical therapist, regular education teacher, special education teacher, principal, special education administrator, both parents, and myself. Nobody looked happy to be there or excited about the task ahead. There seemed to be a defensive tension hanging in the air with the hint of predetermined agendas.

Various professionals droned through their individual reports on the student. Most reported variations on the theme of normal ability that was being compromised by behavioral components typical of ADD/ADHD. The parents were obviously becoming distressed by the recitation of negative comments regarding their daughter's school performance. Finally the parents interrupted with the father defending his daughter as being a "neat kid that was being unfairly beat up" by the professionals. The girl's mother kept apologizing for her daughter's behavior and the challenges and frustrations that it was causing in the school setting. The professionals proceeded to defend their assessment results, and the meeting disintegrated into a "we" and "they" debate. The actual child's needs became lost in the melee of professional posturing and parent emotionality.

The scenario described above is not uncommon. What the situation clearly illustrates is the need for open, honest communication and coordination of services across settings and professionals. Many parents feel that they get placed in the role of coordinating services for their child with ADD/ADHD, a role for which they feel ill-prepared and that they don't want to assume. Thus, it is imperative that school and medical professionals discuss these issues and identify an individual who will be responsible for coordinating assessment and intervention plans across various settings. Regular communication among all parties is needed, and a plan or systematic schedule to monitor progress might be helpful during assessment, initial medication, and early intervention stages. Contact may be less frequent once a child with ADD/ADHD is responding well to interventions—including medication, psychosocial, or academic interventions—and showing steady progress in meeting intervention goals.

Parents are encouraged and expected to participate in the decision-making process regarding their child's physical, emotional, and academic well-being. Parents and professionals share a responsibility to point out a child's needs to each other and to insure consistent understanding.

Building Communication Between Home and School

It is important to create an environment that builds partnerships between parents, teachers, and physicians to better meet the needs of children with ADD/ADHD. One way is through development of a collaborative team, charged with the responsibility to design and implement effective intervention strategies for children with ADD/ADHD. The case example provided an illustration of when a team concept has not been established. In those cases, effective communication is not occurring between team members.

Roadblocks to effective communication between parents and teachers can include the following:
- refusing to acknowledge and accept ADD/ADHD
- communication being problem-driven and only occurring during crisis
- blame being placed on each other or the child with ADD/ADHD
- maintaining a negative focus or outlook toward each other or the child
- making demands or threats
- being defensive
- expecting perfection or quick answers for complex problems
- judging, analyzing, or criticizing instead of jointly problem solving

To overcome the detours of ineffective communication, the following are suggestions to build productive communication between parents and teachers:
- Develop an understanding of each other, the child, and ADD/ADHD.
- Devise a communication system to insure consistent reports to establish a permanent record of strategies and how they worked, and monitor the progress of the communication system on a regular basis.

- Develop a sense of forgiveness—forgive the child and each other when strategies don't work or we experience a bad day.
- Maintain an open mind.
- Keep a sense of humor.
- Share information on ADD/ADHD, ideas, and coping stories.
- Collaborate to find information and answers to problems.
- Know the child's strengths and share positive things about what the child is accomplishing or enjoys.
- Reassure each other.
- Stay focused on the child's best interests and needs.
- Give each other the opportunity to grow and change attitudes.
- Accept that not every parent and teacher will be receptive to new ideas.
- Acknowledge that parents and teachers will not always see things the same way and sometimes have to agree to disagree.
- Learn to view situations objectively rather than arriving at solutions based on emotions.

A Team Approach to ADD/ADHD

This book has consistently stressed the importance of having all individuals who are involved with a child with ADD/ADHD work together. Each member of the team serves an important role in ensuring success for the student. The primary responsibilities for some of the key team members are discussed in the following section.

✔ **The Physician's Role**
Routine physical examinations of children with ADD/ADHD typically document normal results. Pediatricians, child and adolescent psychiatrists, and pediatric neurologists may play an important part in identifying this condition, as well as other possible related conditions. The examination should never be taken for granted. Sometimes it is necessary to conduct medical tests to rule out the possibility of a medical condition that could cause ADD/ADHD-like symptoms. Tests such as chromosome analyses, electroencephalograms (EEGs), magnetic resonance imaging (MRI), or computerized axial tomograms (CT scans) are not used routinely for evaluation of ADD/ADHD and results are generally negative. The neurological components associated with ADD/ADHD are typically referred to as "soft" neurological signs, while positive test results on the previously mentioned

medical tests would suggest "hard" neurological signs substantiating the disorder.

✔ **The Psychologist's Role**

Clinical or school psychologists administer and interpret psychological and educational tests of cognition, perception, and language development (such as intelligence, attention span, visual-motor skills, memory, impulsivity) as well as tests of achievement and social/emotional adjustment. Psychologists and other professionals often integrate data collected from parents and teachers who complete behavior-rating scales about the child in question. Results on such tests can provide important clues as to whether a child's difficulties are related to having ADD/ADHD and/or other problems with learning, behavior, or emotional adjustment.

✔ **The School's Role**

Assessments for ADD/ADHD should always include information about the student's current and past classroom performance, academic skill strengths and weaknesses, attention span, and other social, emotional, or behavioral characteristics. Such information can be gathered through teacher interviews, review of cumulative records, analysis of test scores, and direct observation of the student in class.

✔ **The Administrator's Role**

Administrators need to be trained along with their teachers in learning what ADD/ADHD is and is not. They need to increase their sensitivity and awareness of why these children behave the way they do and what the school should do in terms of implementing appropriate interventions.

Administrators should ensure that teachers have time within their working week to meet with other teachers (particularly at their grade levels) to share ideas and strategies, and plan together. It is also helpful for teachers to observe and even coach each other. Teaming and collaboration require time. Administrators should support collaborative efforts and make this a priority.

Administrators should make sure their staff is trained to understand and accommodate students with ADD/ADHD, especially in techniques focusing on the provision of multisensory instruction. A commitment to

effectively reaching and teaching all students enrolled in a school should include in-service in the following areas:
- cooperative learning
- study/organizational skills
- learning styles
- multiple intelligences (Howard Gardner)
- teacher expectations and student achievement
- tools of technology (computer literacy)
- higher-ordering questioning techniques (e.g., reciprocal teaching)

✔ **The Teacher's Role**

Teacher documentation of specific behaviors exhibited by a child with ADD/ADHD can be very helpful to a diagnostician. Teachers use a number of systems for jotting down notes to themselves to save as "mind joggers" for documentation, reasons for referrals, parent/teacher conferences, and other purposes. Some teachers have a ring of index cards with each student's name on a different card. Whenever something occurs in class that the teacher wants to recall, she jots down the incident and the date on that student's card. Some teachers carry a pad of stick-it notes in their pocket. Later, they transfer all of these notes into a folder they keep on each student. These anecdotal records together with a collection of work samples are very useful sources of documentation.

Frequently, there are questionnaires and rating forms that teachers (or school counselors, school nurses, and other support personnel) are asked to fill out. Typically, the teacher will be asked to provide the following information:
- Describe the child's strengths.
- Describe concerns/child's difficulties.
- Describe current educational functioning levels and performance.
- Identify the testing or school assessments the child has been given.
- Identify the special education services the child receives.
- Identify how the child gets along with other children and adults.
- Identify whether the child has ever repeated a grade.

Even though it is sometimes an inconvenience to complete these forms (especially when teachers are swamped with other paperwork and responsibilities), it is very important to do so. Teachers need to take the time to fill out forms and write their observations in as detailed a manner as possible. This is a professional responsibility that needs to be taken seriously.

✔ **The Parents' Role**

Having witnessed the child in a variety of situations over a number of years, parents have a unique perspective on their child's previous development and current adjustment. Information from parents is usually acquired by interview or through questionnaires completed by parents. The focus is usually on obtaining overall family history, current family structure and functioning, and documentation of important events from the child's medical, developmental, social, and academic history relevant to the assessment of ADD/ADHD.

Guidelines for a Successful Parent/Teacher Conference

Prepare
- Participation by the child with ADD/ADHD and both parents is encouraged. Meet with the teachers as often as needed.
- Develop and bring a list of questions, concerns, and comments in the following areas:
  - ✔ the child's home life, parents' jobs, and the child's interests and hobbies
  - ✔ school policies and programs related to the child, especially any items of specific concern to the child
  - ✔ recent observations of the child's attitude, performance, and behaviors.
  - ✔ examples of current schoolwork
- Anticipate areas of disagreement and develop alternative suggestions.
- Recognize anxiety in other team members; stay calm.
- Appreciate and respect each other's areas of expertise, and keep in mind that each of you is there for the same purpose— to help the child.

Discuss
- Begin the meeting on a positive note by reviewing the child's progress, accomplishments, and successful experiences.

- Discussion should address important items first. Focus should be maintained on the purpose of the meeting and not digress into unrelated issues.
- Include opportunities to ask and answer questions.
- Listen to each other and reassure each other.
- When there are disagreements, explain your objections without accusing or blaming others. Focus on reaching an acceptable solution. Make plans to address remaining problems. If a disagreement cannot be resolved immediately, make a note for later discussion or a subsequent meeting and move on to other items.
- Identify specific actions or ways to help the child and write the ideas down.

Review
- Have the items on your list been covered?
- Are agreements or disagreements resolved?
- Was an action plan formulated?
- Was a date set for a future meeting? Scheduling meetings may be difficult; work with everyone's schedules to establish times so that all can attend the meetings.
- Review the conference with the child, telling him what was discussed and what actions will be taken.

Monitoring
- Are the plans being implemented consistently?
- Are the plans resulting in progress for the child with ADD/ADHD? Classroom observations by parents and teachers can help determine how plans are working and what else needs to be done.
- Take time to congratulate yourself on a task well done!

✔ **The Child's Role**
An interview with the child offers the professional evaluator an opportunity to observe the child's behavior. A personal interaction can also yield valuable information as to the child's social and emotional adjustment, feelings about himself and others, attitudes about school, and other aspects of his life.

✔ **The Team's Role after the Assessment**

Ideally, after all the data has been collected, members of the assessment team should collaborate to discuss their findings. This should lead to a thorough understanding of the child's strengths and areas of need physically, academically, behaviorally, and emotionally. The physician may discuss appropriate medical interventions with the child and parents. The psychologist or other mental health professional may discuss counseling, behavior modification, or social and organizational skills training options. The school may set up classroom interventions to accommodate the child's areas of need in school or may provide special education or related services. Once the initial assessment is completed and appropriate treatment initiated, members of the assessment team should conduct routine follow-up evaluations to monitor the child's progress.

Structure for Collaborative Intervention

ADD/ADHD is a chronic, long-term disorder that requires consistent monitoring on a regular basis to avoid problems. Parents obviously play a key role in encouraging members of the assessment and treatment team to maintain close collaboration. A working relationship with consistent communication will be in the best interest of the child with ADD/ADHD. Coordination of all this, whether it be by a parent or a professional, is no easy task, but the outcome is usually well worth the effort!

When a large number of people are involved in determining the best ways to meet a child's special needs, the process can become cumbersome or lose focus. A model that can be used to help teachers, parents, and other members of the team engage in constructive discussion to generate solutions for the child with ADD/ADHD is explained in the following section. This model can facilitate communication, resulting in reduction of the high level of emotion that frequently surrounds differences of opinion between home, school, or other team members. The steps to accomplish a constructive focus on achieving solutions to problems are listed and explained. These steps are also incorporated into a **Collaborative Intervention Planning Form** on pages 198-199.

Collaborative Intervention Steps

1. Identify Problems and Concerns
2. Identify Potential Solutions
3. Identify Solutions to be Tried
4. Implementation of Solutions (Action Plan)
5. Ongoing Monitoring and Modification of Action Plan

Step 1: **Problem Identification** (Section I of Collaborative Intervention Planning Form)
- ✔ Everyone states perceptions of problems.
- ✔ Problems should be stated in specific terms.
- ✔ Acknowledge perceptions of others.
- ✔ Listen to what others have to say.

Step 2: **Identifying Possible Solutions** (Section II of Collaborative Intervention Planning Form)
- ✔ Brainstorm ideas.
- ✔ Don't be restrictive.
- ✔ Generate a list of possible solutions.

Step 3: **Identifying Solutions to be Tried** (Section II of Collaborative Intervention Planning Form)
- ✔ Evaluate the strengths and weaknesses of each solution considering:
  - • constraints of the classroom.
  - • time and resources required.
  - • needs of the child.
- ✔ Obtain consensus on the solution(s) to be implemented.

Step 4: **Implementation of Solutions (Action Plan)** (Section III of Collaborative Intervention Planning Form)
- ✔ Who will be responsible for each activity?
- ✔ How long will the solutions be tried before reconvening a meeting?
- ✔ How will it be determined that the plan is working?
- ✔ When will the team meet again?

Step 5: **Ongoing Monitoring and Modification of the Plan** (Section III of Collaborative Intervention Planning Form)
- ✔ Obtain ongoing data.
- ✔ Reconvene the team to discuss changes.
- ✔ Decide whether to continue or modify the plan.

Collaborative Intervention Planning Form

Section I	(to be completed prior to team meeting)	
Student's Name:	Grade:	Date:
Completed By:	School:	

1. **Indicate the student's areas of strength.**

Academics:
__ Reading decoding
__ Reading comprehension
__ Written expression
__ Mathematics—recall of basic facts
__ Mathematics—conceptual understanding
__ Rich oral vocabulary
__ Ability to understand complex concepts
__ Spelling
__ Other, please specify_____

Personal Skills:
__ Computers/technology
__ Interacting with peers
__ Memory
__ Leadership skills
__ Interacting with adults
__ Requests help when needed
__ Sense of humor
__ Responds well to praise
__ Demonstrates enthusiasm
__ Other, please specify _____

Comments: _____
_____

Areas of Interest:
__Computers/video games
__Television/movies
__Sports (specify) _____
__Visual arts
__Music (specify) _____
__Volunteer activities (specify) _____
__Other accomplishments _____

2. **Indicate areas of concern that are significantly affecting the student's ability to learn and interact with others at school.**

Academics:
__ Memory
__ Understanding and following instructions
__ Reading decoding
__ Reading comprehension
__ Written expression
__ Mathematics—recall of basic facts
__ Mathematics—conceptual understanding
__ Limited oral vocabulary
__ Ability to understand complex concepts
__ Spelling
__ Other, please specify _____

Behavior:
__ Interacting with adults
__ Motor activity detrimental to learning
   (describe) _____
__ Interrupting, blurting inappropriate
   verbalizations
__ Interacting with peers in class
__ Interacting with peers at lunch and recess breaks
__ Complying with staff requests
__ Transitions between activities or classes
__ Behavior during loosely structured activities
   (assemblies, field trips, etc.)
__ Attendance
__ Other, please specify _____

Organization:
__ Handing in assignments
__ Keeping track of necessary materials
__ Time management
__ Completing tasks
__ Getting started on assigned work

Comments: _____

Section II: Collaborative Intervention Meeting	(to be completed during team meeting)

Date:

Team Members Present:

_____   _____
_____   _____
_____   _____
_____   _____

Possible Solutions/Brainstorming:	Priority
_____	_____
_____	_____
_____	_____
_____	_____
_____	_____
_____	_____
_____	_____
_____	_____
_____	_____

Section III: Action Plan	(to be completed during team meeting)	
1. Strategies to be Implemented:	When	Who
_____	_____	_____
_____	_____	_____
_____	_____	_____
_____	_____	_____
_____	_____	_____
_____	_____	_____
2. How will progress be evaluated?	When	Who
_____	_____	_____
_____	_____	_____
_____	_____	_____
_____	_____	_____
_____	_____	_____
_____	_____	_____
Next Meeting Date/Time:	Place:	

This model to structure collaboration for the team is a process. It is a mechanism for building a relationship between all members of the team to work together for the child with ADD/ADHD. The key to communication in this model is establishing mutual respect and trust by building a caring and supportive relationship.

"Building trust is a process, not an event; time is the key. Simply caring about a child or a parent is all that it takes to start. Listening, regular time together, playing with, validating, respecting and empowering a youngster [parent] will build a positive connection. Children [parents] don't care about how much a teacher knows until they know how much the adults care."

Jerry Moe, Director of Children's Services, Sierra Tucson

Things to Keep in Mind During the Process
- Listen to the perceptions of other participants. Try to understand their points of view.
- Pay attention to what is being expressed emotionally and verbally.
- Avoid exaggerating everything into a crisis.
- Focus on the here and now.
- Avoid blame. This does not solve any problems and interferes with communication.

Collaboration Communication Dos
- Be as specific as possible.
- Be descriptive, not judgmental.
- Be inclusive; make sure everyone gets to express their concerns.
- Acknowledge the perceptions of others.
- Be sensitive to what another person is saying.
- Rephrase what the other person said.
- Foster an open, non-threatening environment.

Collaboration Communication Don'ts
- Avoid blame (e.g., the parent, the child, the teacher).
- Avoid defensiveness: listen without personalizing.
- Avoid judgments.
- Avoid final determination of solutions before all the ideas are generated.

- Avoid using professional jargon.
- Avoid verbal and nonverbal cues that show disrespect.
- Avoid rushing the participants.

Summary

Management of ADD/ADHD requires well-coordinated efforts by a variety of people. Mutual respect, ongoing communication, and sincere commitment to the child with the disorder are absolute necessities for successful intervention. The following graphic presents this balanced approach to diagnosis and management.

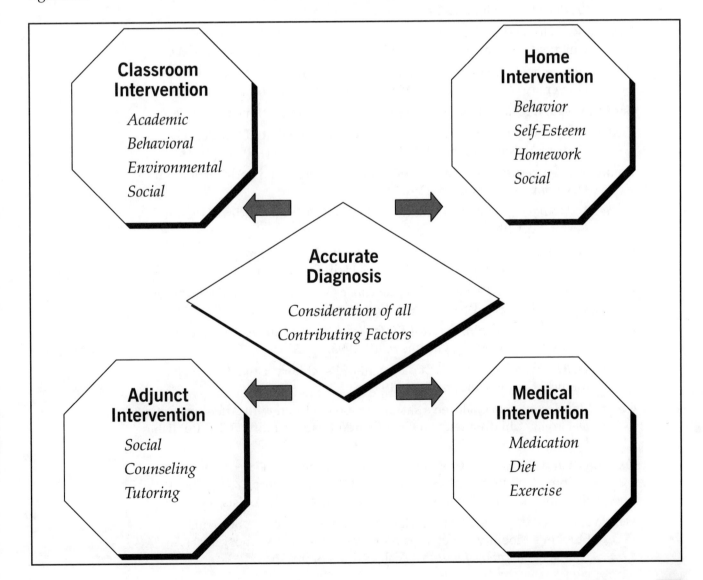

Appendix

Resources

References

"ADHD myths result in delayed treatment," *Advance for Speech-Language Pathologists & Audiologists*, Vol. 10, No. 25, June 26, 2000, p.6.

American Psychiatric Association, *Diagnostic and Statistical Manual of Mental Disorders*, fourth edition, American Psychiatric Association, Washington, D.C., 2000.

Barkley, R.A., *ADHD and the Nature of Self-Control*, Guilford, New York, 1997.

Barkley, R., *Attention Deficit Hyperactivity Disorder: A Handbook for Diagnosis and Treatment*, The Guilford Press, New York, 1990.

Barkley, R. "Home situations questionnaire," Department of Psychiatry, University of Massachusetts Medical Center, Worcester, Mass., 1989.

Barkley, R., "School Situations Questionnaire," Department of Psychiatry, University of Massachusetts Medical Center, Worcester, Mass., 1989.

Barrett, Susan, *It's All in Your Head*, Free Spirit Publishing, Minneapolis, 1992.

Biederman. J and S. Faraone, "Attention Deficit Hyperactivity Disorder," *The Harvard Mahoney Neuroscience Institute Letter,* Vol. 5(1), 1996, pp. 1-3.

Brandt, R., "Powerful Learning," Association for Supervision and Curriculum Development, Alexandria, VA 1998.

Caine, R., *Making Connections: Teaching and the Human Brain*, Addison Wesley, Boston, MA 1994.

Carbo, M., Dunn, R., & Dunn, K., *Teaching Students to Read Through Their Individualized Learning Styles*, Prentics Hall, Englewood Cliffs, NJ, 1986.

Clark, L., *SOS Help For Parents: A Practical Guide for Handling Common Everyday Behavior Problems*, Parents Press, Bowling Green, KY, 1985.

Collins, M. and S. Benjamin, *Survival Kit for Teachers and Parents*, 2d ed, Goodyear Books, ScottForesman, Glenview, Ill., 1993.

Conners C.K., "Conners Scales," Department of Psychiatry, Duke University Medical Center, Durham, N.C., 1991.

Council for Exceptional Children's Task Force on Children with Attention Deficit Disorder, "Children with ADD: A Shared Responsibility," CEC Publishing Reston, VA, 1992.

Dawson, P. and R. Guare, "Attention Disorders' Interventions for Adolescents Helping Children At Home and School: Handouts from Your School Psychologist," National Association of School Psychologists, 1998.

Della Valle, J., et al., "The Effects of Matching and Mismatching Students: Student's Mobility Preferences on Recognition and Memory Tasks," *Journal of Educational Research*, Vol. 79.5, 1986, pp. 267-272.

Dendy, Chris, *Teenagers with ADD: A Parents Guide*, Woodbine House, Inc., Bethesda, STATE, 1995.

Downs, B., *ADD and Problem Solving:A Model For Home School Physician Partnerships*, School District of Elmwood, Brookfield, Wis., 1998.

Dunn, R. & Dunn, K., "Dispelling Outmoded Beliefs About Student Learning," *Educational Leadership*, Vol. 44.6, 1987, pp.55-61.

Ford, Martin, *Motivating Humans*, Sage Publications, Newbury Park, CA, 1992.

Goldstein, S. and M Goldstein, *A Parents Guide: Attention-Deficit Hyperactivity Disorder in Children*, Neurology Learning and Behavior Center; Salt Lake City, Utah, 1995.

Goldstein, S. and M. Goldstein, *Attention-Deficit Hyperactivity Disorder: The Current State of the Field*, Neurology Learning and Behavior Center, Salt Lake City, Utah, 1993

Greenough, W. T., "Cerebellar Synaptic Plasticity: Relation to Learning Versus Neural Activity," *Annals of the New York Academy of Science*, Volume 627, 1991, pp. 231-247.

Hannaford, C., *Smart Moves*, Great Ocean Publishing Co., Arlington, VA, 1995.

Hocutt, A. et al., "Issues in the Education of Students with Attention Deficit Disorder: Introduction to the Special Issue," Exceptional Children, Vol. 60(2), 1993, pp.103-106.

Hunter, Madeline, *Mastery Teaching*, T.I.P Publications, Es Segundo, CA, 1982.

Jensen, Eric, *Brain-Based Learning*, Turning Point Publishing, Del Mar, CA, 1996.

Jensen, Eric, *Completing the Puzzle: The Brain-Based Approach*, Turning Point Publishing, Del Marr, CA, 1996.

Jensen, Eric, *The Learning Brain*, Turning Points Publishing, Del Mar CA

Jensen, Eric, *The Learning Brain*, The Brain Store, Inc., San Diego, 1995.

Jensen, Eric, *Teaching with the Brain in Mind*, Association for Supervision and Curriculum Development, Alexandria, VA, 1998.

Journal of American Academic Child & Adolescent Psychiatry, Vol. 35 (9), 1996, pp. 1193-1204.

Kimura, D., "Male Brain, Female Brain: The Hidden Difference," *Psychology Today*, November, 1989.

Kimura D., "Sex Differences in the Brain," *Scientific American*, September, 1992, pp. 119-125.

Kosslyn, Steven, *Wet Mind*, Simon & Schuster, New York, 1992.

Kuhn, H. G., "More Hippocampal Neurons in Adult Mice Living in an Enriched Environment," *Nature*, Vol. 38, 1997, pp. 493-495.

"Laying the groundwork for understanding brain-related disorders of attention," *Advance for Speech Language-Pathologists & Audiologists*, Vol. 9, No. 32, August 9, 1999, p.21.

Levine, Melvin D., *Developmental Variation and Learning Disorders*, Educator Publishing Service, Inc., Cambridge and Toronto, 1993.

Lozanov, Georgi, "On Some Problems of the Anatomy, Physiology, and Biochemistry of Cerebral Activities in the Global-Artistic Approach in Modern Suggestopedagogie Training," *The Journal of the Society for Accelerated Learning and Teaching*, Vol. 16.2, 1991, pp. 101-116.

Marey, D., *How to Own & Operate an Attention Deficit Kid*, CHADD, Roanoke, VA, 1993.

McCarney, S.B., *Attention Deficit Disorders Evaluation Scale: Home Version*, Hawthorne Education Services, Columbia, Mich., 1989.

McCarney, S.B. and A. Bauer, *The Parents Guide to Attention Deficit Disorders*, Hawthorne Education Services, Columbia, Mich., 1990.

McCarney, S. B., *The Attention Deficit Disorders Intervention Manual*, Hawthorne Educational Services, Inc. Columbia, Mich., 1989.

McCarthy, Michael, *Mastering the Information Age*, Jeremy Tarcher, Los Angeles, 1991.

McGinnis, E. and A.Goldstein, *Skills-Streaming in Early Childhood*, Research Press Co, Champaign, Ill., 1990.

Meese, R., *Strategies for Teaching Students with Emotional and Behavioral Disorders*, Brooks/Cole Publishing Company, Pacific Grove, Cal., 1996.

Moir, Anne & Jessel, D., *Brainsex*, Dell, New York, 1991.

Nadel, L., "Varieties of Spatial Cognition: Psychological Considerations," *Annals of the New York Academy of Sciences*, Vol. 608, 1990, pp. 613-626.

Parker, H., *The ADD Hyperactivity Handbook for Schools*, Impact Publications, Plantation, Fl., 1992.

Phelan, T., *All About Attention Deficit Disorder*, Child Management Inc., Glen Ellen, Ill., 1989.

Physician's Desk Reference, 52nd ed., Medical Economics Data Production Company, Montavie, N.J., 1998.

"Practice Parameters for the Assessment and Treatment of Children, Adolescents and Adults with Attention Deficit/Hyperactivity Disorder," *Journal of American Academy of Child and Adolescent   Psychiatry*, Vol. 36(10), October 1997.

Rief, S., *How to Reach and Teach ADD/ADHD Children*, The Center for Applied Research in Education, West Nyak, N.Y., 1993.

Rosenfield, I., *The Inventions of Memory*, Basic Books, New York, 1988.

Shinsky E.J., *Students with Special Needs: A Resource Guide for Teachers*, Shinsky Seminars, Lansing, Mich., 1996.

Web Sites

The Brain Store
www.thebrainstore.com

Child Development Institute
http://childdevelopmentinfo.com/disorders/medications.shtml

Organizations

ADDA: Attention Deficit Disorders Association
P.O. Box 543
Pottstown, PA 19464
484-945-2101
www.add.org

CESD: Council of Educators for Students with Disabilities, Inc.
9801 Anderson Mill Rd., Suite 230
Austin, TX 78750
512-219-5043
www.504idea.org/about_us.html

CHADD (Children and Adults with Attention Deficit/Hyperactivity Disorders)
8181 Professional Place, Suite 150
Landover, MD 20785
800-233-4050
www.chadd.org

Family Resources Center on Disabilities
20 E. Jackson Blvd, Room 300
Chicago, IL 60604
800-952-4199
www.frcd.org

26-05-9876543

Resources

Appendix

Silver, H.F., et al., *Teaching Styles and Strategies*, Thoughtful Education Express, Woodbridge, N.J., 1996.

Sprenger, M., *Learning & Memory*, Association for Supervision and Curriculum Development, Alexandra, VA, 1999.

Sousa, D., *How the Brain Learns*, The National Association of Secondary School Principals, Reston VA, 1995.

Sylwester, Robert, *A Celebration of Neurons: An Educators Guide to the Human Brain*, Association for Supervision and Curriculum Development, Alexandria, VA, 1995.

Taylor, M., "Evaluation and Management of Attention-Deficit Hyperactivity Disorder," *American Family Physician*, Vol. 55 Num. 3, 1997, pp. 887-894.

Teeter, P.A., "Attention-deficit hyperactivity disorders: A psychoeducational paradigm," *School Psychology Review*, Vol. 20(2), 1991, pp. 266-280.

Teeter, P.A. and P. O'Brien-Stewart, *ADD and Problem Solving Communication: A Model for Home School-Physician Partnerships*, School District of Elmbrook, Brookfield, Wis., 1998.

Ullman, R.K. et al., ACTeRS Teacher Form, 2nd ed. Institute for Child Behavior and Development, Champaign, Ill., 1991.

United States Dept. of Education & Rehabilitation Services, "Clarification of Policy to Address the Needs of Children with Attention Deficit Disorders Within General and/or Special Education," Washington D.C., 1991.

Weill, M., *Attention Problems: Strategies for Parents and Teachers*, National Association of School Psychologists, 1998.

Weinstein, R., "Avoid misdiagnoses: Use ADD/ADHD specialist to insure correct ID of students with attention disorders," The Special Educator, Vol. 15(8), 1999.

"What prevents children with ADHD from getting the treatment they need?" *Advance for Speech-Language Pathologists & Audiologists*, October 23, 2000, p. 20.

Wlodkowski, R., *Enhancing Adult Motivation to Learn*, Josey-Badd, San Francisco, 1985.

Woodward, D. and N. Biondo, *Living Around the Now Child*, Charles E. Merrill Publishing Company, Columbus, Ohio 1972.

Wree, A., "Sexes Differ in Brain Degeneration," *Anatomy and Embryology*, Vol. 160, 1989, pp.105-119.

Zeigler-Dendy, C.A., *Teenagers with ADD: A Parents Guide*, Woodbine House, Bethesda, MD; 1995.

Copyright © 2001 LinguiSystems, Inc.